MIGRAINE

Not Just Another Headache

First published in 2016 by Currach Press
23 Merrion Square
Dublin 2, Ireland
www.currach.ie

ISBN: 978-1-78218-886-5
Set in Freight Text Pro 10/13
Cover and book design by Helene Pertl | Currach Press
Printed by ScandBook AB

MIGRAINE

Not Just Another Headache

Edited by Marie Murray

Compiled by Patrick Little & Audrey Craven

CONTENTS

FOREWORD

Dr Marie Murray

The title of this book, *Migraine: Not Just Another Headache*, points to the classic misconception of migraine as a bad headache rather than the complex, disabling affliction that it is. The book itself is a unique collation of the finest expertise from some of the foremost migraine professionals in Ireland, North and South. It is a book that guides the reader through all the aspects of migraine that anyone who suffers from migraine, or lives with a sufferer, would wish people to know.

And 'suffer' is the word for what migraineurs do. Migraine is not just a headache. It is not just a bad headache. It is not even an excruciating headache. It is, as most of the authorities in this book note, a significant neurological disorder that requires careful management and that intrudes on every aspect of the migraineur's life. Migraine affects the lives of 12–15% of the population – that's more than half a million people in this country suffering from what most of the writers in this book agree is a frequently undiagnosed, misdiagnosed or delayed diagnosed condition. We know what happens when people suffer in silence and when they feel alone and misunderstood. It is psychologically alienating, personally distressing, physically disabling, socially isolating, and practically intrusive on family life and relationships. It may impact on educational attainment, vocational selection, workplace relationships and career advancement.

Distinguished by its pain and unpredictability, this book shows how migraine can strike anywhere, anytime. Holding the sufferer's life to ransom because of its devious, episodic, capricious visitations, the threat of migraine is intimidating. This is one of the most oft-cited distresses of the condition, because how can you organise your life when whatever you have planned can be sabotaged? How can you keep friends if you must constantly cancel on them at short notice? How can you advance in your career when you may have to absent yourself at critical times? How can you sustain relationships when your partner, your children, your extended family may be 'let down' at no notice, when it seems that you can never be present for what matters to them? And how can you have good self-esteem when others see you as 'unreliable' and confuse the disorder with you?

As you read the chapters in this book you will see how migraine, that never-welcome guest, may stay an hour, or two, or twenty-four or seventy-two, and may even make a quick return visit just when you thought it had left. Or it may send a warning signal: an advance aura or notification of its intention, sufficient to put fear into the heart of experienced migraineurs. Attacks can include feelings of irritability or confusion, thirst, fatigue, sensitivity to light and sound, stomach upset, flashing lights, zigzag patterns before the eyes, pins and needles on one side of the body. Speech may be slurred and there may be loss of coordination – and oh what an irony that a migraineur might appear to be drunk when the last thing a migraineur wants is alcohol. Migraineurs are probably the least likely people to be 'under the influence', given that alcohol is one of the classic triggers for an attack.

Of course the first step towards any solution is knowledge. Knowledge about migraine gives the sufferer the power to combat it. You have to know what you are up against before you can deal with it. Knowledge is what this book provides. You open the book to uncover the combined expertise of clinicians across all aspects of migraine, with each chapter addressing another dimension. This Migraine Association of Ireland (MAI) book is a multidisciplinary specialist migraine consultation for readers. For example, Patrick Little, the CEO of the MAI, tracks developments internationally to ensure that those who contact the Migraine Association are directed to psychoeducational interventions, clinical services, legislative information and disability rights. His chapter provides an important overview on migraine with key statistical data and analysis of the impact of migraine on people's lives. His advice to migraine sufferers is clear: 'get a diagnosis, get the right treatment, get the right support, take control' – the perfect preface to a book that guides the sufferer on how to do so.

In her chapter 'A life living with migraine', Audrey Craven brings us into the real, raw lived experience of the condition as only a migraineur can. Inspirational in how she turned her personal experience of migraine self-management into founding the Migraine Association of Ireland, she has engaged in relentless national and international neurology patient advocacy work ever since, developing services and negotiating at the highest level on behalf of sufferers. Audrey Craven's story is powerful. Her message is realistic but upbeat: 'migraine is common, disabling and treatable.' Treatable. That is the key word. That is the word to hold on to, as she encourages 'those who suffer in silence and isolation to seek the information and support they require to get their lives back'. Nobody represents hope better than Audrey Craven does.

Paediatric Neurologist Dr Deirdre Peake's chapter on 'Migraine in Children' alerts us to something that may be new to many parents – that is how common, yet under-diagnosed, headaches in children can be. In ordinary life we tend not to think of children and headaches, and they rarely complain of them. Dr Peake explains how migraine in children may be 'abdominal', taking the form of the tummy ache we so associate with children when they are upset. And who would have thought that approximately 25% of adolescents suffer weekly headaches? When adolescents withdraw they may have very good reason to do so, especially if they are undiagnosed suffers of migraine. For any of us who work with young people this is another possibility to always keep in mind.

Professor Martin Henman's chapter on 'Going to the Pharmacy' leads us through the minefield of medications for migraine. He helps us to understand the delicate balance between the benefits and risks of medication for migraine and alerts us to the impact of excessive drug use to alleviate pain which, ironically, may cause additional problems in the form of rebound or medication overuse headache (MOH). This is also an important chapter in informing and reassuring us about the role of drugs and other treatments for migraine, as he leaves no possibility of migraine relief unattended to.

Nor is any possibility left unexamined in Professor Orla Hardiman's new insights into migraine from the neurological perspective. With the rigour of a researcher, the exactitude of an academic and the compassionate curiosity of the clinician, her chapter is a must-read for absolutely up-to-date information about migraine in all its manifestations. One intriguing nugget in her account is the work she reports on that suggests that what have previously been perceived to be external triggers may actually be part of the migraine event. My sentiment on finishing her chapter, rich with its necessary density of neurological detail, is appreciation for the expertise in this country, lightly worn and generously given, so that whatever treatments may emerge from research Irish migraineurs will be the first to benefit.

General Practice is the cornerstone of medicine. We tend to admire and rely on our GPs. They are almost always the first physician we call upon, which is why Dr Paddy Daly's chapter provides a special view on headaches in general practice and how to get the most from your GP consultation and from medication if you are a migraineur. Ultimately, he says, 'migraine becomes about three times more common in women than in men' and so he also shines an important light on women and migraine which both women and men will benefit from by reading.

Clinical Director of the Cork University Migraine Clinic Dr Eddie O'Sullivan's chapter is another trove of information on the multidisciplinary approach to migraine management in specialist migraine clinics, and he provides a clear and essential outline of migraine management in sport. Sportspeople will welcome his advice on the most effective acute therapies for treatment of exercise-induced migraine. Everyone needs to read his treatment recommendations following a concussive head injury and study his section on post-traumatic headaches – rugby players especially take note!

Julie Sugrue, who is a clinical specialist physiotherapist, focuses on the role of physiotherapy in the management of migraine, particularly in the management of the neck pain associated with migraine. Her chapter helps us understand the extent, if any, to which neck pain and migraine may be related, and she draws the distinction between those who will benefit by physiotherapy and those who will not. In her open, honest and direct style the benefits and contraindications for physiotherapy are revealed, concluding with practical online resource information for readers.

Migraine costs the European economy €27 billion annually in reduced productivity. The World Health Organisation (WHO) put this figure at up to £140 billion globally and according to the Migraine Association of Ireland, migraineurs miss up to an average of 4.5 days of work annually at a cost of €252 million to the Irish economy. This startling information is given by Dr Caoimhín MacMaoláin, Associate Professor of Law at Trinity College, Dublin, who addresses the role of law in protecting chronic migraine sufferers in their employment. This is a significant chapter. Analysing current law, he queries whether anti-discrimination directives based on disability might apply to those occasions when migraine attack symptoms temporarily 'disable' the migraineur. When this happens, he asks, would aspects of the relevant legislation be applied to accommodate and to protect the sufferer of chronic migraine symptoms? No employer, employee or human resource department wishing to understand current legislative protections and responsibility can ignore this chapter.

In my own 'Psychology and Migraine' chapter I explore some of the psychological implications, family interactions, therapeutic interventions and lifestyle adjustments of chronic illness that clinical experience suggests may assist in migraine management, while the final chapter in this book provides a range of tips for living with migraine that have been devised by the Migraine Association of Ireland Helpline Team. A key tip given is to read this book because, as the team advise, 'with the right information, support, treatment and understanding, the majority of migraineurs can bring their condition under control, reducing the frequency and severity of attacks, thereby living a full life'.

So why read this book? Admittedly it takes some dedicated reading, because it respects the reader's capacity to study and absorb the clinical terminology and dimensions of this neurological disorder. But if you suffer from migraine, live with a migraineur or have family or close friends with migraine, then you know personally what a chronic, incapacitating, unpredictable and crippling condition migraine can be. If this is your acquaintance with migraine, then I believe that this book is important for you. It will not only provide you with additional information, but it will validate you or your experiences of sometimes feeling helpless, frustrated, fearful, angry or awed in the face of the chronic suffering endured by migraineurs and those who care about them, especially in the period before diagnosis and in the early stages of lifestyle adjustment to the condition.

If you are not acquainted with migraine then this book is equally for you. This is because, as you can see from this foreword, the common misconception that migraine is 'just a headache' or 'a bad headache' is an idea that has added to the distress of sufferers due to how exceptionally misunderstood they and their condition can be.

If you are a professional working in physical or mental health then this book is a must, as it brings you into the lived reality and cutting-edge scientific thinking on migraine. Professionals working with children will benefit by understanding the symptoms of migraine, which might mimic behavioural or other problems. Adolescents whose developmental stage is already often misunderstood may be suffering additional challenges to their age and stage with undiagnosed migraine, or have other neurological needs. It is important for us to understand that the so-called irritability of adolescence might sometimes be the aura of a migraine attack.

Psychologists, psychiatrists, psychotherapists, family therapists, clinical nurse specialists, social workers, school guidance counsellors, cognitive behaviour therapists, life coaches and others will appreciate the potential co-morbidity of migraine, mood disorder and depression and will welcome this understanding extending out into mental health discourses. Educationalists and teachers will welcome the multidisciplinary perspectives on students who suffer from migraine. Human Resource professionals will value the insights into the needs of the migraineur to extend policy and flexible working practices in order to increase the individual's productivity while supporting them during periods of temporary 'disability'. Staff relations can be improved by there being organisational understanding and acceptance of migraine when it is a disability.

In childhood, in adolescence, in adulthood, in men and in women in ordinary everyday life, migraine manifests itself in many guises and disguises, and this book outlines them for you. In summary, it looks at migraine prevalence, its impact, trends, triggers and treatments; the experience of sufferers; multidisciplinary approaches; the role of the physician, the GP, the neurologist, the pharmacist, the physiotherapist, the psychologist. It advises about management in relationships, the family, the home, the school, the sports centre, the workplace. It gives crucial information from neurology and from specialist migraine clinics about pain management, migraine in children, migraine in adolescents, migraine in school, migraine in the workplace, and the legislation to support people in educational and employment contexts.

This is a broad, expert-based sweep that cannot but inform thinking and policy at national level and internationally. Buy it, read it, put it in your local community, in your library, in your surgery, in your practice, in your clinic. Put it in your school, your college, your student union and disability support services. Give it to your family, your friends, your colleagues at work and to anyone who would welcome understanding that migraine is not just another headache.

INTRODUCTION TO MIGRAINE

Patrick Little

Patrick Little has been CEO of the Migraine Association of Ireland (MAI) since 2008. He is a Board member of the European Headache Alliance and also a Board member of the Neurological Alliance of Ireland, the umbrella organisation for neurological patient groups in Ireland. He is a member of the National Council of the Disability Federation of Ireland, and also an active member of IPPOSI – The Irish Platform for Patients' Organisations, Science & Industry. Prior to working with the MAI he lived in Scotland for thirty years, where he worked in the NGO sector as Scottish Development Manager for Young People's Services for a large mental health charity.

INTRODUCTION

In this opening chapter I will give an overview of migraine and the impact it has, and set the scene for other contributors to cover different aspects of migraine in more detail later in the book.

As the name of the book suggests, migraine is not 'just another headache'. It is a severely debilitating, complex and disabling condition which affects an estimated 12–15% of the population (over 500,000 people in Ireland).

It is a recognised neurological disorder (i.e. a disorder of the brain, spine and the nerves that connect them) which is now ranked the sixth most disabling disease in the latest World Health Organisation (WHO) Global Burden of Diseases study published in 2013 and the fourth amongst women. Severe migraine attacks are classified by the WHO as among the most disabling illnesses, comparable, during an attack, to dementia, quadriplegia and active psychosis. According to the WHO, tension-type headache and migraine are the second and third most prevalent medical disorders on the planet. Over 30,000 people in Ireland suffer from chronic migraine, which means they experience headache on fifteen days or more every month.

Typical characteristics of migraine are that:

o The pain is pulsating, generally but not always on one side of the head.
o It is usually aggravated by physical activity.
o It is accompanied by sensitivity to light or noise, and nausea or vomiting.
o It normally lasts 4–72 hours.
o Around 20% of migraine sufferers experience visual disturbance, which is called aura.
o In extreme cases symptoms can mimic a stroke with temporary paralysis down one side of the body.

Despite some regional variations, migraine is a worldwide problem which affects people of all races, ages, income levels and geographical areas. Migraine is a highly individual condition in that apparent triggers and responses to treatments differ from person to person.

Migraine is 3:1 more common in women than men, usually occurring during the most productive years, and studies have shown that 60% of migraine is hereditary. This is important to know, as children of migraineurs are therefore potentially more at risk of inheriting the 'migraine gene'. An estimated 10% of children suffer from migraine and in children the split is 50:50 male:female.

Migraine costs the Irish economy an estimated €252 million annually and the European Union €26 billion in a combination of workdays lost and reduced productivity. These figures do not include the cost of medical treatment of migraine.

Studies have shown that on average it takes six years to get an accurate diagnosis for migraine. During this time the wear and tear on people's lives can be significant, with relationships and work severely impacted. In many cases, by the time people contact the Migraine Association of Ireland for help they are very troubled, feeling weary, isolated and hopeless, often not feeling in control of their lives and desperately in need of help.

THE BURDEN AND IMPACT OF MIGRAINE

'I'm not okay. I have lost it all – sports, husband, friends, job, independence and the will to live ...'
— Extract taken from a Migraine Association Helpline email and reproduced with the permission of the author.

The burden of migraine and other primary headache disorders should not be underestimated because the impact on the lives of people who suffer can be extensive, going much beyond the headache disorder itself. There is considerable evidence from Irish statistics, based on a recent major European Quality of Life study, that people with migraine face particular challenges as a result of their condition. These include dealing with ongoing pain, stigma, poverty, social isolation and exclusion, unemployment, underachievement, relationship difficulties, and experiencing related mental health problems.

Some headlines from the Irish data from this European study carried out in 2010 show:

Headache frequency
In the previous thirty days prior to taking part in the study:

o 17% of participants had headache on 15 days or more.
o Of these 61% had headaches lasting 3 hours or more.
o 63% were taking medication on 15 days or more.

Most bothersome headache
o 37% lasted 1–3 days.
o 8% lasted 4–6 days.
o 48% described it as 'bad' and 45% as 'very bad'.
o 62% could not do some things and 31% could do nothing at all during this headache.
o 76% felt sick and 24% were actually sick.
o Light bothered 77% and noise 94%.

IMPACT QUESTIONS

Migraine impacted on several aspects of people's lives:

Education
o 14% did less well or gave up early.

Career
o 28% did less well or took an easier job.
o 31% reported reduced earnings as a result of their headaches.
o 42% felt employers and colleagues did not accept or understand.

Family and friends
o 88% felt family and friends understood and accepted their headaches.
o 46% avoided telling other people.

In the last three months
o 77% could not go to work on 1–3 days because of their headache.
o 38% could do less than usual at work on 5 days or more.
o 35% could not do any household work on 5 days or more.
o 42% could do less than half on 5 days or more.
o 41% missed family, social or leisure activities on 5 days or more.
o 62% who had children were prevented from caring for them.
o 22% of partners missed social activities.

Quality of life
o 29% were very dissatisfied or dissatisfied with their health.
o 16% were very dissatisfied or dissatisfied with their ability to perform daily living activities.
o 12% were very dissatisfied or dissatisfied with their personal relationships.
o 16% had little or no energy for everyday life.

Depression and anxiety
o 23% felt tense or 'wound up' a lot or most of the time.
o 34% felt they were slowed down very often or nearly all of the time.
o 10% still enjoyed the things they used to only a little or not at all.
o 18% got frightened feelings quite often or very often.
o 24% may not take quite as much care about their appearance as they did.
o 20% can't laugh and see the funny side of things quite so much now.
o 42% felt restless very much or quite a lot.
o 35% have worrying thoughts a great deal or a lot of the time.
o 46% look forward with enjoyment to things rather less or definitely less than they used to.

The reported co-morbidity of migraine with depression and anxiety was further backed up by a study carried out in 2012 by a student at the School of Medicine and Medical Science at University College Dublin who found that 26% of respondents were diagnosed with depression, almost 20% with anxiety and 13% with panic attacks.

Migraine not only impacts on the sufferer but also on those people in contact with them – family, friends, employers, colleagues and health professionals. To begin with, many migraineurs begin to self-medicate with 'over-the-counter' medications purchased in pharmacies and other outlets. If these do not work they start to increase the amount they are taking, leading many to develop a new kind of headache called 'Medication Overuse Headache'. This will be covered in detail in later chapters.

General Practitioner training on headache and migraine is disproportionately low given the statistics on suffering and incapacitation arising from migraine. For example, during their professional education General Practitioners reportedly receive an average of four hours' training on headache even though it is one of the most common issues with which they will be presented in their future practice. It is most important then, and a leading aim of the Migraine Association of Ireland, to increase the knowledge and awareness of health professionals in order to provide both earlier and improved responses to migraine sufferers. There is a Health Professional section on the Migraine Association of Ireland website (www.migraine. ie) where health professionals can access the International Headache Society criteria for diagnosing migraine, in addition to information on all types of headache disorders.

NEUROLOGY CLINICAL PROGRAMME

Currently the Health Service Executive (HSE) is developing a National Neurology Clinical Programme which includes a Care Pathway on Headache. The mission of the programme is to develop a framework to support provision of a multidisciplinary, high-quality and responsive service to all patients suffering from neurological conditions in a timely and efficient manner, from first contact with a GP to treatment at a specialist headache centre.

To meet the needs of both current and indeed future patients with neurological conditions, the vision of the programme is to develop services which are safe, responsive and able to offer all patients support with respect to:

o Early and appropriate assessments, diagnosis and equitable management.
o Integrated Care Pathways across the continuum of care.
o Development of properly resourced services to support the patient journey.

The proposed Care Pathway on Headache maps a patient journey and provides guidelines based on best practice and a multidisciplinary approach to headache care. This will result in patients having access to early intervention and quality treatment at a primary care level. This should also mean that people are not being unnecessarily referred on to specialist headache clinics where there are currently long waiting lists as a result of inappropriate referrals. People with more complex headache needs will then have quicker access to Consultant Neurologists, Specialist Headache Nurses, Psychology support, Headache Physiotherapists, etc.

YOUNG PEOPLE AND STUDENTS

Reasonable Accommodations
To facilitate and provide a level playing field for students with disabilities, the State Examinations Commission (SEC) has devised what are called 'Reasonable Accommodations'. Getting through exams can be stressful in its own right and, for students living with migraine, the worry about attacks during exam time can lead to added pressure.

Students should request a confirmation letter from their GP/Neurologist stating that they have been diagnosed with migraine. Both the SEC and the school will need this to proceed to an application for Reasonable Accommodations, which should be submitted in the year prior to examinations. The following is the current official information from the SEC on applying for Reasonable Accommodations, along with their contact details:

Applying for Reasonable Accommodations
o If necessary these can include a request for a special centre within the school for the candidate to sit the examination on their own.
o You must have a letter from the student's GP/consultant before approaching the State Examinations Commission.
o Please be aware that the student may apply to have a tape recorder to record answers if they are unable to write.

o In the event that the student cannot sit the examination at the scheduled time they can sit it later on that date provided they have prior approval, are supervised by a member of the school authority, and have had no contact with other candidates or anyone who may have had sight of the question paper, or knowledge of its contents. Candidates may not, however, take an examination on a later date under any circumstances.

Should the student be well on the day and have no need to avail of the special centre the Reasonable Accommodations Office should be notified. This can be done on the day of the examination and an email will suffice.

The current contact number for the Reasonable Accommodations Office is 090-644 2782/ 3/ 4/ 5/ 6 and their email is sec.specialneeds@examinations.ie.

The DARE Programme
Disability Access Route to Education (DARE) is a third-level alternative admissions scheme for school-leavers whose disabilities have had a negative impact on their second-level education. DARE offers reduced points places to school-leavers who as a result of having a disability have experienced additional educational challenges in second-level education.

AHEAD
AHEAD, the Association for Higher Education Access and Disability, is an independent non-profit organisation working to promote full access to and participation in further and higher education for students with disabilities, and to enhance their employment prospects on graduation.

AHEAD has sections for people who are looking to go to college, for those already in college, for people looking for work, and for teachers, lecturers and other professionals who work in the college environment. There are links for employers too, and tips on how to approach an employer regarding disability issues, as well as legal information. They have links to several organisations and websites that might offer further tips and information.

FIVE KEY HINTS TO A BETTER LIFE

o Get informed – Increase your own knowledge. The Migraine Association of Ireland (MAI) has a website, www.migraine.ie, with extensive information on all aspects of migraine. Keep a migraine diary which records all aspects of your life for a period including what you eat, sleeping patterns, weather, use of medications and frequency and severity of the pain. The diary can help you identify and avoid your trigger factors. MAI also produces quality information leaflets on various aspects of migraine.

o Get a diagnosis – Find a sympathetic GP who has knowledge of and interest in headache issues and bring your completed diary with you. This will substantially increase your chances of getting a good diagnosis and appropriate treatment.

o Get the right treatment – There are two main types of medical treatments for migraine, acute intervention and preventative treatment, which will be covered in detail later in the book. If the treatment you receive from your GP does not improve your situation, ask for a referral to a specialist headache clinic. There are five in Ireland and they are free – all that is required is a letter from your doctor.

o Get the right support – Dealing with migraine can be a lonely, isolating journey. Get information for your friends, family, employers and work colleagues. MAI runs a Helpline (1850 200 378) and a nurse advice line.

o Take control – Build resilience and self-management skills by attending MAI seminars and self-help groups (more on MAI in the next chapter). A User Satisfaction Survey carried out by MAI at the end of 2015 found that a staggering 46% of those questioned scored 10/10 on how their migraine/headache had impacted on their overall quality of life prior to contact with MAI services. Following attendance at MAI events this was considerably reduced, with 76% of people reporting a positive impact on their management skills and a much improved quality of life.

COMPLEMENTARY THERAPIES

Complementary therapies are defined as techniques that are not part of the medical school curriculum but may be seen as complementing mainstream medicine. For several years now there has been a dramatic increase in the numbers of people using complementary techniques to treat migraine as the concept of integrated medicine has become more acceptable.

Many Irish migraine sufferers report benefits, and at least some relief, through therapies such as:

o Acupuncture
o Biofeedback
o Reflexology
o Meditation
o Mindfulness
o Cognitive Behavioural Therapy
o Yoga

The conventional medical profession has viewed this growth with some scepticism. However, MAI believes that if the individual experiences some benefits from using safe complementary practices, then their appropriate use is to be supported for that individual. MAI would, however, also advise that the authenticity of the qualifications of any practitioner a person intends to attend are checked out to ensure that they are affiliated to the relevant national bodies or associations and that the practitioner's previous history of treating people with migraine and other headache disorders has been ascertained. Many complementary treatments are free from side effects, but some are contraindicated with certain illnesses and medications, so it is advisable to consult your doctor in advance. Herbal medications are discussed further in the pharmacy chapter of this book.

Some doctors will have trained in complementary approaches and many more encourage their use. Scientific research continues into complementary treatments for migraine and it is accepted that certain treatments have some benefits for some people. Currently there is a study in progress between Dublin City University and the only Outpatients Neurology Centre in Northern Ireland on the use of Neurofeedback (i.e. a form of biofeedback or training for the brain using technology which shows the brain working) for the treatment of migraine.

Finally, don't give up hope. There are new devices increasingly coming on the market which are showing promising results and a new group of specific migraine medications in the later stages of clinical trials which should be available in the next few years. While migraine can be a very debilitating condition there is no evidence to suggest that frequent attacks of migraine can cause any long-term damage to the brain and in most, but not all, cases, migraine reduces with age.

REFERENCES

o Vos et al., 'Global, regional, and national incidence, prevalence, and years lived with disability for 301 acute and chronic diseases and injuries in 188 countries, 1990–2013: a systematic analysis for the Global Burden of Disease Study 2013', *The Lancet*, Volume 386, Issue 9995, pages 743–800, 22 August 2015. [http://www.thelancet.com/journals/lancet/article/PIIS0140-6736(15)60692-4/abstract]

o 'The Cost of migraine and other headaches in Europe', Berg, L., Stovner, L. J., *European Journal of Neurology*, 2005;12(Suppl 1):59–62, June 2005.

o Olesen, J., Gustavsson, A., Svensson, M., Wittchen, H. U., Jönsson, B., on behalf of the CDBE 2010 study group and the European Brain Council, 'The economic cost of brain disorders in Europe',

European Journal of Neurology, Volume 19, Issue 1, pages 155–162, January 2012.

o Yusop Md, Little, P., Costello, J., Ryan, D., 'Migraine and Mental Wellness', School of Medicine and Medical Science, University College Dublin, 2012.

2

A LIFE LIVING WITH MIGRAINE & THE WORK OF

THE MIGRAINE ASSOCIATION OF IRELAND

Audrey Craven

Audrey Craven, a lifelong migraineur, is committed to sharing hard-won experience of migraine self-management in the hope of improving the quality of life for all those affected.

In 1994, Audrey's journey inspired her to found the Migraine Association of Ireland, leading to better recognition of the impact and burden of living with migraine. This role evolved into national and international neurology patient advocacy work. She serves as immediate Past President of the European Federation of Neurological Associations and the European Headache Alliance. Audrey was the only patient representative on the European Commission's 'Healthy Brain; Healthy Europe' scientific board for European Month of the Brain 2013.

'Finding the key', as depicted in the Migraine Association of Ireland's logo above, is as individual as a thumbprint. My personal journey reflects the despair and subsequent empowerment of one severely affected by migraine. I hope it will encourage those who suffer in silence and isolation to seek the information and support they require to get their lives back. Remember: migraine is common, disabling and treatable. The editor of this book, Dr Marie Murray, said 'I am not my migraine' when she addressed a public migraine information seminar years ago. This is so true and her message inspired many of us to lead full lives and do what we can to reduce the burden. I trust this book will help you and yours.

As a child, I suffered from what I now know to be abdominal migraine. This gradually progressed to severe one-sided headaches, vomiting and diarrhoea from my twenties onwards. Migraine attacks lasting two to three days occurred five or six times a year, deteriorating to three or four times a month in my thirties. My three young children tiptoed around the house because I couldn't bear noise or light. I was fortunate to have a supportive family as I struggled to function. There is no doubt that the burden is determined by your ability to function during an attack – mine is like a power cut and 'Not just another headache'!

Many doctors mistakenly believe that patients have unrealistic expectations of a magic bullet or miraculous cure when they seek treatment. In fact, all they require is a clear explanation and an empathetic approach to the management of this complex condition. Various studies have demonstrated that the typical 'severe headache patient' usually explores numerous avenues in search of treatment. Google the word 'migraine' on the Internet and thousands of remedies are offered to the enquirer. Many are from quacks and charlatans ready to exploit those who are so desperate that they will consider unlikely and unorthodox remedies in their quest for relief.

I sought medical help, and also tried numerous quacks in search of a cure. I have vivid memories of ingesting a foul herbal decoction, formulated by a traditional healer, every day for three months – with no beneficial effect whatsoever! In reality what patients require most is reliable information and support on their journey to 'finding the individual key' to better self-management. This enforces the 'Accept and Act' theory which many now recommend as an important step on the journey from despair to personal empowerment.

Unfortunately, I was hospitalised frequently due to dehydration for what seemed to most people to be 'just a headache'. There was little or no information available in pre-Internet Ireland. I made a vow to the good Lord that if I ever got some form of self–management, I'd do something to improve the quality of life for others. Migraine did not *ruin* my life, but it certainly *ruled* it!

I read an article written by a world-leading migraine expert in London and made an appointment in 1990. He diagnosed basilar migraine and told me, if it was any comfort, that I was one of the worst cases he'd ever seen! The development of Triptan medications has changed our lives and the subcutaneous version (because it is so rapidly absorbed) certainly changed mine. I joined the then British Migraine Association and found their quarterly newsletter to be a lifeline. At last someone truly understood. I followed their advice to keep a migraine diary, identify triggers, look at maintaining a healthy lifestyle, and slowly reclaimed my life. This involved regular eating, sleeping, and drinking fluids – in other words living life defensively. It seems the migraineur's brain likes regularity.

Everyone gets headaches; so when a friend suggested that the next time I got one I should go for a walk, I realised she had no understanding of how disabling a migraine attack can be. The fact that I needed to be in a darkened room, close to the bathroom, had not occurred to her despite our friendship of many years. She also had no idea that the risk of such frequent attacks was ever-present in my mind. This fear arising from the unpredictability of attacks – better known as the interictal (time between attacks) effect – can lead to anxiety and depression.

With the lack of understanding among the general public, it's no wonder that the pan-European study 'EUROLIGHT' on quality of life issues found that 47% of respondents avoid telling other people about their migraine. In the same study however, 88% of people surveyed felt that close friends and family understood the burden of coping with an invisible illness.

Many migraineurs don't want to talk about their attack once it is over, with most not consulting their GP, mistakenly believing there is nothing to be done, so it remains a hidden disorder. They may have witnessed a family member (as there is 60% genetic predisposition) suffer in silence and isolation, so they do too. Those who do consult may not be treated appropriately, as most doctors receive training in ruling out a 'sinister' headache only and very little training on migraine and other primary headache disorders.

However, finding an interested GP is a very important step towards better management and improved quality of life. There is no 'test' for migraine, as the diagnosis is based on good case history taking. Keeping a headache diary (available from MAI) can help ensure a person gets the best from a medical consultation and a more accurate diagnosis.

The societal and economic impact of migraine and other headache disorders is possibly unquantifiable. The reality of everyday life for sufferers is that normal function is interrupted by migraine episodes at irregular and unpredictable intervals. This can impose severe limitations on their daily lives, whether at school, at work or during leisure time. How do you measure the loss of treasured family and social occasions? The EUROLIGHT study results reflect the impact on family life, with 62% of people with children saying they were prevented from minding them and 22% of partners saying they missed social events.

Equally important are the lost days in the workplace, as well as lost opportunities by not applying for promotion for instance, and the resultant economic consequences. Again, the EUROLIGHT results demonstrated the impact on career decisions, with 28% of respondents saying they did less well or took an easier job as a result of living with migraine.

Despite increasing recognition of migraine as a complex neurological disorder, it is apparent that many patients still feel that it is not being sufficiently recognised as a debilitating condition, resulting in stigmatisation and the erroneous perception of a 'neurotic malingerer'! This is especially evident in the case of workplace prejudice, where migraineurs have a fear of being seen as work-shy, unreliable or lacking commitment if they take time off during migraine episodes.

In order to give yourself the best opportunity of managing migraine in your workplace I would recommend carrying your medication on your person at all times and, if possible, try to rest in a quiet, darkened room when migraine hits. Most people will be able to return to work and be productive members of staff if this is facilitated. Try to give deadlines a few days to spare, for instance Wednesday instead of Friday. Also build a 'favour bank' at work – in other words, develop a relationship of mutual support and educate your colleagues at work who can potentially cover for you when you need time out and vice versa.

MIGRAINE ASSOCIATION OF IRELAND

'Whilst seeking the cure MAI provides the care'

By 1994, I was able to manage sufficiently to call a public meeting; hence the Migraine Association of Ireland (MAI) was born. Those early volunteers who worked tirelessly had a vision of a world where the condition would be recognised, taken seriously and managed appropriately.

One of the most valuable roles for patient organisations lies in sifting and filtering indiscriminate tranches of information, particularly on the Internet, by working in tandem with the scientific community and other partners to ensure that information on conventional and complementary therapies is reliable, readily available and up to date.

A patient organisation can provide practical help, support and information on how to deal with migraine at work or at school. It can provide promotional material for employers and school authorities and so forth to raise their levels of awareness, leading to better understanding and mutually beneficial strategies for dealing with problems or avoiding them entirely.

The importance of 'peer-to-peer' support cannot be overemphasised as studies demonstrate that peer-to-peer led education and self-management support courses have better outcomes. Reports indicate that patients 'know' more when information is received from health professionals, but actually 'do' more when information is shared by trusted peers.

The primary purpose of the Migraine Association of Ireland (MAI) is to alleviate the burden of migraine and other headache disorders by:

o Providing accurate, reliable information and support.
o Helping people identify early warning signs and trigger factors.
o Promoting healthy living and lifestyle issues.
o Creating a forum for peer-to-peer support.
o Increasing awareness of migraine and other headache disorders.
o Advocating for better services.
o Encouraging research.

These aims are achieved by providing a range of services including:

o A free helpline 1850 200 378 (ROI) 0844 826 9363 (N.I.).
o Specialist nurse advice line.
o A website with a public, health professional and children's sections, www.migraine.ie.
o Public information seminars.
o Support groups.
o Outreach events for employers and employees.
o Accredited health professional training events.
o Producing the MAI BrainStorm magazine with up-to-date world news and treatments.
o Monthly e-zine newsletters.
o Quality information leaflets on all aspects of migraine.
o Advocating for specialist headache clinics – the five headache clinics in Ireland came about from campaigning and support from MAI.

Over twenty-two years on, the staff and Board of the Association are proud to be regarded as 'the most active and forward looking Headache Patient Association in Europe' (Professor Jes Olsen, former President of the European Brain Council).

The services provided by MAI to the patient and medical community in Ireland have been acknowledged many times, including:

o In 2003 our information pack for health professionals earned the 'Patient Association of the Year' award.

o The MAI website won the award for Best Use of Information Technology at the Irish Pharmaceutical Healthcare Awards in 2006 and now has over 40,000 hits annually.

o In 2009 MAI won the 'Best use of Technology Award' at the Irish Healthcare Awards for the design of an electronic migraine diary.

o 2015 saw MAI win the first GSK Ireland Impact Awards for 'demonstrating excellence in community health'.

In recognising the need for co-operation between MAI and relevant health professionals in the provision of best practice services to patients, I also realised there was significant scope for joint endeavours in the area of advocacy, policy promotion with government departments and business interests with other neurological groups in Ireland. This mutuality prompted the establishment in Ireland of an alliance between the various lay associations representing people with neurological conditions.

The Neurological Alliance of Ireland (NAI) is an umbrella organisation for twenty-eight patient organisations. It is difficult for any government to talk to twenty-eight individual organisations, but by working together and delivering a unified message in partnership with the scientific and other relevant stakeholders some progress has been made. NAI has already had an enormous impact and influence on government policies and funding programmes and has produced policy papers that have been implemented. Similar organisations have been and are being established in many countries.

EUROPEAN HEADACHE ALLIANCE (EHA)

Quite apart from the extensive co-operation that can exist within national boundaries, between the relevant patient associations and health professionals there is an established and growing level of liaison and mutual international support between lay associations themselves, particularly between European countries. Some of the liaison is formalised on a Europe-wide basis through the European Federation of Neurological Associations (EFNA), which combines European umbrella bodies of neurological patient advocacy groups. In order to promote the cause of headache at European level I founded the European Headache Alliance (EHA) in 2006. It was officially launched in Brussels at the European Parliament by Nobel Laureate John Hume back in 2006. EHA now represents twenty-five headache patient organisations across the continent.

A hugely important function of national and European organisations is to provide information to policy makers and the public at large, by raising awareness of the condition and by encouraging research. These roles are probably best illustrated by reference to the development and operation of services provided by the Migraine Association of Ireland over the years and its successes to date. Patient organisations have learnt that political persuasion is most readily achieved by learning from the success of campaigns, for example those of cancer research and heart disease, and their methodologies, and from sharing best practice between countries.

It took years of advocacy and argument to have migraine and other headache disorders acknowledged and recognised as a leading cause of disability. It is now generally accepted that migraine is the most common neurological condition in the world, affecting an estimated 600 million people worldwide. It is therefore more common than epilepsy, asthma and diabetes combined; but it does not yet have the recognition or service provision that many less common disorders attract. In fact, it is the least publicly funded of all neurological illnesses relative to its economic impact.

To address this the EHA launched the 'What's Under the Hat?' campaign, designed to raise awareness of headache disorders amongst the general public across Europe. The campaign also creates a platform to bring stakeholders together to influence policy makers.

Evidence-based arguments, repeated by patient organisations and the relevant health professionals, are the most effective means of persuading key opinion leaders such as those formulating policies, devising budgets and ordering priorities. The patient voice as a trusted third party is increasingly central for all decision makers. A major benefit which is anticipated from international alliances (apart from increased lobbying potential) is the sharing of expertise and information, and the expansion of research opportunities beyond national patient groups.

Despite the growing body of research into headache and migraine disorders, there is huge scope for further research and the role of patients. Clinical trials are less likely to fail at advanced stages if patients have been involved at an early stage, making it financially prudent to do so.

Policy makers attach great importance to preventative therapies and services, so research in this field is vital, as is scientific-based research on the impact and burden of migraine on individuals and the community. The role of patient organisations in providing data and real-life patient experience for such studies is now seen as central to the health agenda in Europe. The MAI and EHA are considered key stakeholders in headache discussions and collaborate on a number of national and European initiatives.

EMPOWERMENT

My personal journey of reaching out in a time of despair was a process of empowerment. Many years ago my then ten-year-old niece encapsulated this in the slogan: 'Don't suffer migraine in the dark, let the Migraine Association of Ireland help you move into the light!' It is hard to keep in mind that migraine is common, disabling and treatable when caught in the vortex of numerous attacks. Feelings of guilt prevail as we try to think what we have done or not done to provoke this attack. Knowing that I was not alone on this journey is what motivated me to continue this advocacy work. Accepting that we have a brain disorder is a major part of learning to cope and self-manage.

Achieving a work/life balance is an ongoing battle, but being kinder to ourselves certainly goes a long way to achieving it.

The growth in the development of well-organised, properly resourced and interlinked patient organisations should be viewed positively by the scientific community and can be regarded as a worthwhile and valuable resource in the shared goal of improving treatments, services and beneficial research in the field of migraine and other headache disorders. Exciting, innovative new therapies are on the horizon, so the future looks brighter.

Remember, the character and pattern of migraine can change at any stage of your life. Sudden onset over the age of fifty should be investigated. It is comforting to note that the burden usually reduces with age, but many productive years are blighted by this debilitating neurological disorder.

Use this book to help take control of your migraine and please know that you are not alone. Seamus Heaney (my favourite poet) put it beautifully: 'Even if the hopes you started out with are dashed, you must keep hope alive!'

For further information and links to national patient organisations please contact the following:

Migraine Association of Ireland – www.migraine.ie
European Headache Alliance – www.europeanheadachealliance.org
European Federation of Neurological Associations – www.efna.net

3

MIGRAINE: NOT JUST ANOTHER HEADACHE

Orla Hardiman

Orla Hardiman was appointed as the first full Professor of Neurology in Ireland by Trinity College Dublin in 2013, where she is now Academic Director of the Biomedical Science Institute, and heads the Academic Unit of Neurology. She is a Clinician Scientist and Consultant Neurologist at the National Neuroscience Centre of Ireland at Beaumont Hospital, Dublin, where she was also Clinical Director of the first Migraine Headache Clinic developed in Ireland. Orla has become a prominent advocate for neurological patients in Ireland and for patients within the Irish health system generally. She is co-founder of the Neurological Alliance of Ireland, and Doctors Alliance for Better Public Healthcare.

INTRODUCTION

Migraine is a relatively common but frequently misdiagnosed condition that affects approximately 12–15% of the population. It manifests as a unilateral (one-sided) throbbing headache that occurs periodically and normally lasts 4–72 hours. Diagnosis is based on the presence of a constellation of symptoms discussed in this chapter.

ADVANCES IN THE PATHOPHYSIOLOGY OF MIGRAINE

Recent studies in neurophysiology and neuroimaging have demonstrated that migraine is a neurological (brain and nervous system) disorder characterised by episodic disruption of brain activity. This is a very important and recently recognised principle, as the original understanding of migraine was that it was primarily a disorder of the vascular (blood vessels) system.

Our understanding of migraine has been significantly enhanced by improvements in imaging technology (where we can see the brain in action), and there is now definitive evidence that blood vessels do not constrict during an acute episode of migraine. Rather, as demonstrated by what are called positron emission tomography (PET) images taken during acute migraine attacks, migraine is associated with activation in the brainstem, one of the oldest parts of the brain from an evolutionary perspective. This activation persists after the treatment of pain, and is not present between attacks.

Measures of brain activation between migraines also show that the brains of migraineurs behave differently to non-migraineurs in between migraine attacks. For example, migraineurs do not respond to some patterned visual stimuli (i.e. pictures that provoke a response) in the same way as people who do not have migraine. The neural networking underlying these differences is not very well understood. However, there have been significant advances in fundamental research around migraine, and new treatments will undoubtedly be developed that are based on these differences.

There are several different types of migraine. The International Headache Society classification of headache can be found at: http://www.ihs-headache.org/ichd-guidelines.

Migraine can occur with or without aura. Aura refers to a range of neurological disturbances: visual disturbance such as seeing zigzag lines, spots, flashing lights; sensory disturbance, confusion, etc., that precedes the headache. The aura is self-limiting, and typically lasts 15–20 minutes. The headache associated with aura is usually less severe than that in migraine without aura. Migraine without aura was often previously called 'common migraine', and migraine with aura was called 'classical migraine'.

MIGRAINE WITHOUT AURA

At least five attacks where headache attacks last 4–72 hours and has at least two of the following characteristics:

o Unilateral location (on one side).
o Pulsating quality (throbbing).
o Moderate or severe intensity.
o Aggravation by routine physical activity (most people just need to lie still).

During the headache, at least one of the following:

o Nausea and/or vomiting.
o Phonophobia (sensitivity to sound).

MIGRAINE WITH AURA

At least two attacks which have at least three of the following four characteristics:

o One or more fully reversible aura symptoms.
o At least one aura symptom (as described above) develops gradually over more than four minutes, or two or more symptoms occur in succession.
o No aura symptoms last more than sixty minutes.
o Headache follows aura within less than an hour; it may also begin before or at the same time as the aura.

MIGRAINE WITH TYPICAL AURA

The way to diagnose migraine with typical aura is if it fulfils criteria for migraine with aura, including all four criteria below. One or more symptoms of the following types:

o Homonymous visual disturbance, which is loss of vision towards one side in each eye, but which is the result of disturbance in the brain and not in the eyes.
o Unilateral paraesthesias (one-sided tingling, pins and needles) and/or numbness.
o Unilateral (one-sided) weakness.
o Aphasia (impairment of speech) or unclassifiable speech difficulty.

It is estimated that around 25% of migraineurs experience aura symptoms and around 1% experience the aura symptoms with no subsequent headache. There are people who experience migraine both with and without aura. There is no difference between migraine with aura and migraine without aura with regard to the efficacy of anti-migraine drugs.

EPISODIC TENSION-TYPE HEADACHE

Episodic tension-type headaches are defined when people have at least ten previous headache episodes but less than 180 headache days per year; where no evidence of other disease which could cause headache could be found; where the headache lasts thirty minutes to seven days; and where at least two of the following pain characteristics are present:

o Pressing, non-pulsating quality.
o Mild or moderate intensity.
o Bilateral location (the pain is in both sides of the head).
o The headache is not made worse by routine physical activities.

Both of the following are also true:

o No nausea or vomiting.
o No sensitivity to noise (phonophobia) or to light (photophobia) or just sensitivity to one of these.

TRANSFORMED MIGRAINE /CHRONIC DAILY HEADACHE

This is a prolonged headache syndrome that at first seems like a typical migraine, but subsequently becomes a milder but more prolonged headache syndrome. This is the kind of migraine that is managed and benefits by early treatment of migraine attacks, and long-term medication (prophylactic therapy) with anti-migraine drugs.

BASILAR MIGRAINE

This is a rare form of migraine that includes symptoms such as loss of balance, double vision and fainting. During the headache some people lose consciousness and it is more common in young women.

HEMIPLEGIC MIGRAINE

This is another rare but severe form of migraine where temporary paralysis occurs, usually on one side of the body. It often begins in childhood and there is usually a strong family history.

OPTHALMOPLEGIC MIGRAINE

Ophthalmoplegic migraines, also known as ocular migraines, are a very uncommon type of migraine headache in which the eye region is the focal point of the pain. The headache can be accompanied by temporary eye muscle weakness or paralysis, which may persist for days to weeks after resolution of the headache. The first occurrence of ophthalmoplegic migraine typically takes place during childhood. Intermittent attacks may persist into adulthood.

MEDICATION OVERUSE HEADACHE (MOH)

MOH is a chronic headache which evolves as a consequence of overuse of over-the-counter and prescription medication. As the body becomes accustomed to medication, a lowering of the blood levels of analgesics (painkillers) can be associated with a rebound headache (headaches caused by taking pain relief for headache), which drives the person to take more medication. This leads to a vicious cycle of taking medication to relieve a headache that is itself caused by the medication. The only cure for MOH is complete withdrawal, generally recommended under the supervision of a GP.

MEDICAL EVALUATION OF HEADACHE

People presenting with a typical history of migraine and a normal physical examination do not require any further investigations. However, key factors that must be considered in eliciting a history of headache are:

o Headache onset (or when headache/s began).
o Location and duration of pain.
o Frequency and timing of attacks, including triggers.
o Pain severity and quality.
o Associated features.
o Aggravating, precipitating and ameliorating factors (anything that makes it worse, that triggers or relieves the problem).
o Family history and past medical history.
o Physical and neurological examinations.

DIAGNOSTIC ALARMS IN HEADACHE EVALUATION

There should be no evidence of other diseases which could cause headache.

o History, physical and neurologic examinations that do not suggest another headache type.
o History and/or physical and/or neurologic examinations that suggest another disorder, but is ruled out by further investigations.

There are a number of important features that should alert the physician to an alternative diagnosis, which are as follows:

o Onset or beginning of headache syndrome after fifty years of age.
o Sudden onset headache – no warning of headache.
o Accelerating pattern of headache or change in the nature of an existing headache.
o New onset headache in cancer or HIV.
o Systemic illness.
o Focal neurological signs.
o Papilloedema (swelling of the optic nerve).

OTHER FEATURES OF MIGRAINE

While most people associate migraine with sensitivity to light, nausea, and vomiting, there are many other features associated with migraine that often go unrecognised. These include a reduction in gastric functioning, changes in temperature regulation and other visceral (internal organs of the body, such as heart, lungs or abdomen) functions. In children, migraine can manifest as a syndrome of periodic abdominal or stomach pain, or as episodic vomiting (see later chapter on children).

A significant minority of people also suffer from vestibular symptoms (impairment of balance) as part of their migraine. It is increasingly recognised that episodic vertigo can be a migraine variant. The association between vestibulopathies (for example Méniére's disease, a disorder of the inner ear which can cause hearing problems, dizziness, loss of balance, vertigo and other problems) and migraine has been poorly recognised until recently.

More complex migraine can include hemisensory loss (loss of sensation on one side of the body), hemiplegia (one-sided paralysis), confusion and on rare occasions, loss of consciousness.

MIGRAINE TRIGGERS AND ASSOCIATED FEATURES

Migraine attacks can be divided into different phases (above). Not all of these phases will be experienced by everyone. Many people with migraine can identify triggers that are associated with its development. Missed meals, late nights, weather, stress, menstruation, certain foods and alcohol are many of the features that people describe as contributing to their migraine and usually a combination of these are seen as triggering their migraine.

However, there is an intriguing body of recent work that questions the authenticity of external migraine triggers. This work suggests that perceptions of these triggers are actually part of the migraine event. For example, a study of participants who reported that their migraines could be triggered by light failed to demonstrate this in a research setting. This has led to speculation that these patients notice light in the initial or prodromal phase and that this is why they associate light as a trigger. Other work has suggested this with other reported triggers, including some types of food (such as chocolate), stressful events and so forth, all of which could be the start of the migraine disruption of neurological function rather than external triggers. In other words the migraine episode has already begun when the so-called 'triggers' are noticed, so that they don't cause it but are the start of it. It is an interesting possibility.

Migraine is also associated with other symptoms, including a high incidence of exaggerated skin sensitivity (cutaneous allodynia). Migraineurs often describe increased scalp and skin sensitivity around the eyes when they are combing their hair, shaving, showering or wearing glasses during a migraine attack. Evidence suggests that earlier Triptan treatment for migraine reduces the development of allodynia or pain sensitisation.

MANAGEMENT OF MIGRAINE

Migraine is a primary headache disorder – there is no other known structural or external cause. As a result, drug treatments for migraine may be acute (symptomatic) or preventative (prophylactic). Patients with frequent severe headaches often require both approaches. As the complex mechanisms underlying migraine are discovered, new classes of drugs are undergoing development both to limit attacks and prevent recurrences.

For example, there is evolving evidence that migraine is associated with activation of primary sensory neurons ('meningeal nociceptors') in a part of the nervous system known as the trigeminal ganglion, which release a protein called calcitonin gene-related peptide (CGRP) from their projecting nerve endings located within the lining of the brain (meninges). This work has led to novel and promising strategies for the treatment of migraine using CGRP antibodies against this pathway, and new drugs based on this are expected to become available in the next few years.

ACUTE TREATMENT

Acute treatments attempt to relieve or stop the progression of the attack, or to abort it once it has begun. Acute treatment is appropriate for most attacks but should be used a maximum of 2–3 days a week, unless under the supervision or direction of a doctor. Analgesics and Triptans are established as standard therapies for symptomatic management of the headache associated with migraine.

ANALGESICS

Analgesics are painkillers. They do not act on the cause of the pain, but work by reducing the person's perception of it, effectively numbing the pain-affected area. Analgesics are a favoured and effective treatment for many migraineurs. Primary ones used by migraineurs would include:

o Aspirin
o Paracetamol
o Non-steroidal anti-inflammatory drugs (NSAIDS).

ANTI-EMETICS

The main purpose of anti-emetics is to combat nausea and sickness. They have no direct impact on migraine, but they can be used in two particular circumstances:

o If nausea is a major part of the attack. This is a symptom in the vast majority of migraine attacks, and like the headache symptom, it too should be treated. Suppositories are a good option for anyone who experiences severe nausea or vomiting.
o Anti-emetics also aid the absorption of other medications into the system. During a migraine attack, absorption is slowed dramatically and this reduces the impact that analgesics can have. Taking a mild anti-emetic about fifteen minutes before an analgesic will increase the chances that the analgesic will be effective.

TRIPTANS

Triptans (or 5-HT agonists) are the migraine-specific, prescription-only drugs that became available in the 1990s. A major breakthrough in migraine treatment, these medications target specific groups of serotonin receptors in the brain that are known to be closely involved in migraine attacks. There are six Triptan drugs available in Ireland at the time of publication. These are Almogran (Almotriptan), Frovex (Frovatriptan), Imigran (Sumatriptan), Zomig (Zolmitriptan), Naramerg (Naratriptan) and Relpax (Eletriptan).

The main advantages of these medications are that they are fast-acting, can be effective even if taken up to two hours into an attack and are beneficial in up to 80% of cases. In addition to tablets, other formulations are also available, depending on the Triptan. Orally disintegrating tablets (dissolves on the tongue), nasal sprays and injectable forms are often faster acting and preferable for those who suffer from nausea. Anti-emetics do not need to be taken with Triptans.

While all of the Triptans have proven to be effective, there are some differences in typical side effects, speed of action and headache recurrence rate. Analysis of the drugs has concluded that due to different way people respond to chemicals (biochemical individuality), an individual's response to a Triptan cannot be predicted. If one Triptan fails, another within the class may well succeed.

PREVENTATIVE THERAPIES FOR MIGRAINE

Preventative treatment is used in an attempt to reduce the frequency and severity of anticipated attacks. A number of medications in use for other conditions have been found to be of value in treating headache, albeit in different dosages, and are now commonly prescribed for migraine. These include:

o Beta Blockers – originally designed to combat angina and high blood pressure.
o Anti-Convulsants – originally used to prevent seizures in patients with epilepsy.
o Anti-Depressants – affect the serotonin receptors.
o Calcium Channel Blockers – high blood pressure.
o 5-HT Antagonists – interfere with the action of seratonin.

However, it is important to realise these medications will not prevent attacks altogether and will not cure the underlying cause. They are usually prescribed in one of five circumstances:

o If the person suffers from more than two or three attacks per month which are treated with acute remedies.
o If attacks are particularly severe or disabling and do not respond well to acute treatments.
o To break the cycle of attacks, enabling treatment of attacks at a later stage with acute treatments.
o If attacks follow a regular pattern (for example around the time of menstruation).
o In the case of forms of migraine such as basilar (additional symptoms include loss of balance) or hemiplegic migraine (additional symptoms include partial paralysis on one side).

Preventatives are taken daily for a period of 9–18 months, starting at a low dose and slowly building up every four weeks. While they rarely prevent attacks altogether, their success rate is about 50–60%. However, all prophylactic (preventative) medications have latency of 8–12 weeks. This means that people experience side effects of medications prior to experiencing any benefit, which means that people may give up taking them before they have had a chance to work and so lose out on potentially beneficial medication for their migraine.

OTHER THERAPIES

Botulinum Toxin (Botox)
There is evidence that treatment with botulinum toxin can improve chronic daily headache in a subset of patients. Treatment should be reserved for those who have not benefited from conventional preventative agents, and who are not overusing analgesics. Limitations of treatment include cost, and the fact that the effects of botulinum toxin decline after 2–3 months, and repeated treatments are necessary.

Greater Occipital Nerve Block
There is limited evidence that a block of the greater occipital nerve (a spinal nerve that stimulates the scalp at the top of the head)

can improve chronic migraine. However, there is a lack of placebo-controlled data (that is, testing at the same time with a matched group of people with a drug that has no physical effect to see if the result is psychological rather than from the drug) in support of this intervention, with recent publication of at least one negative double blind study (a study in which nobody at all knows who is taking the 'real' drug or the 'fake' or placebo drug) in 2015.

Neuromodulatory Therapies

With increased recognition that migraine is primarily a neurological event, a number of neuromodulatory (changing nerve activity through electrical stimulation) agents are under development, with varying degrees of success. Invasive treatments such as greater occipital nerve stimulation have not been successful. Novel studies using transcranial (through the skull) electrical stimulation and vagal nerve stimulation (sending electrical impulses) are currently under investigation.

CONCLUSION

Migraine is recognised as a disabling neurological condition, with specific clinical characteristics. There have been considerable advances in our understanding of migraine, with the pace quickening over the past ten years. Treatment strategies should be instituted as early as possible after the onset of pain to prevent central sensitisation, which may otherwise limit how well the treatment works.

At present, it should be possible to control migraine effectively in the majority of patients using the treatment types currently available. Further understanding of the pathophysiology (study of the condition and changes) of migraine will lead to the development of new and more specific therapeutic options for migraine prevention in the future.

4

GOING TO THE PHARMACY

Martin Henman

*Martin Henman is Associate Professor in the Practice of Pharmacy
in Trinity College, Dublin. He is a registered pharmacist and is a
member of the Steering Group of the Irish Institute for Pharmacy
which is responsible for CPD. In 2006, he was presented with the
Provost's Teaching Award for the excellence of his contribution in
TCD. He has published on Pharmaceutical Care, Cancer, Palliative
Care and Medicines use in the Elderly. He is researching optimising
medicines and supplement use in the Intellectual Disability Supplement of TILDA. He is a fellow of the European Society of Clinical
Pharmacy.*

INTRODUCTION

Community pharmacies are a front-line service run by Primary Care
professionals who practise in almost every town and village in Ireland
and are easily accessible without an appointment. Interestingly, they
spend around a quarter of their time dealing with patients' questions
not directly related to medicines.

Pharmacists and their staff are ready and able to help and advise
sufferers of migraine. Their primary concern is the well-being of their
patients. To do this it is essential that a fruitful patient–pharmacist
relationship is established. If patients set out to get the best out of
their pharmacy it will help them to keep control of their migraine and
to get the best out of their medication. New information and advice

is continuously being made available about migraine and the medications and supplements used to treat it, so it is good to talk regularly to the pharmacist to see if any of it is relevant to you.

If you are in a pharmacy and have a concern about the standard of the advice or service that you have received, raise it with the pharmacist. If you do not want to do this, you should speak to the Migraine Association of Ireland (MAI), or you can contact either the Irish Pharmacy Union or the pharmacy regulator, the Pharmaceutical Society of Ireland.

Community pharmacists exercise a duty of care to those who come to ask for their help and advice. They have four main areas of responsibility:

o Assisting patients and prescribers with the use of prescription medicines and medical devices.
o Providing and advising about the use of non-prescription medicines and supplements.
o Assessing and advising patients about symptoms.
o Primary and Secondary Health Promotion and advice about health and lifestyle.

Communication between patients and pharmacists is crucial if medication use is to be optimised. In dealing with migraine, the use of medication to treat an attack or to prevent attacks means that the topic of migraine medication is complex. The active ingredient of any medication or drug can bring significant benefits, but only if used precisely as intended, and the potential side effects can be effectively managed if they are understood and recognised. This balance between the benefits and risks of a medication must be at the heart of the conversation between a patient and their pharmacist.

Not everyone who works in a community pharmacy is a pharmacist but the other staff may also be qualified to help with medicines, either as a pharmacy technician or as counter assistant or healthcare assistant. This team complements and supports the work of the pharmacist, and the procedures of the pharmacy operation ensure that when necessary a patient with complex needs will be referred to the pharmacist.

INFORMATION ABOUT MEDICATION

Prescriptions are requests from a prescriber, often the person's GP, to a pharmacist to provide a medication for the patient. Prescriptions name the medication and usually indicate how it is to be taken. Pharmacists are required to check these and other details to satisfy themselves that the prescription and the medication are in the best interest of the patient. Since the prescription does not tell the pharmacist what the medication is to be used for, this, and some other information, may be sought from the patient at the first dispensing (preparation, labelling, recording and transfer) of the prescription. Once the pharmacist has this information they can determine the suitability of the medication, provide it to the patient and meet their professional obligations. This process serves as a check in the steps leading to medicine use and protects patients from misadventures. In this way, pharmacists exercise a duty of care towards patients receiving medications.

The old saying that 'knowledge is power' can be applied to medications; knowing about them and their role in the treatment of a condition is a first step to controlling that condition and living as full a life as possible. Important pieces of information are:

o The name of the medicine – both the active ingredient (drug name) and the brand name or manufacturer.
o For what purpose it is used.
o How, as well as how often, it should be used.

It is vital that whenever a change is made to medications it is discussed with the pharmacist, together with any other changes to the patient's conditions or circumstances. Each time a prescription is dispensed in a pharmacy a record is created and associated with this dispensing. The record, which the pharmacist may keep, notes significant clinical issues, so that when the patient hands in another prescription those notes are available as a guide. This helps to provide continuity of care, which is important for an effective and safe health service.

The vast majority of medications come with a patient information leaflet. This is a very valuable document – it has been approved by the Health Products Regulatory Authority (the Medicines Regulator) and covers, in a clear and consistent way, all of the relevant information about the product and its use. It is worth reading through the leaflet and keeping it in a safe place so that you can consult it if you feel you need to do so.

There are more than ten drugs and forty products of prescription medication authorised for use in the treatment of migraine. Both prescribers and patients assume that all medications are always available; but unfortunately this is not the case, as particular products, strengths or formulations may be temporarily unavailable in Ireland. Information about shortages may not be readily accessible and is constantly changing, so patients may only find out that a drug is unavailable when they present their prescription at the pharmacy.

Because this is a worldwide problem, the Irish Pharmacy Union collates as much information as it can to help pharmacists and patients. Community pharmacists will do their best to obtain a supply of a medication for a patient and pharmacists work together so that, usually, they are successful. Sometimes an equivalent preparation may have to be provided and for some medications it may be necessary for the pharmacist to consult information compiled by the Health Products Regulatory Authority to identify a suitable preparation.

ADHERENCE

In the first couple of weeks of taking medication, it is worth thinking through the likely impact on your daily activities. If taking your medication is going to be difficult because of the number of doses that have to be taken at different times in the day, tell your pharmacist to see if you can find ways to reduce the burden or to schedule them more conveniently.

By working with the pharmacist to adapt both the medication taking and your lifestyle in a way that suits you, you are more likely to be able to stick to it in the long term – healthcare professionals call this adherence, and good adherence ensures increased effectiveness of medication.

Similarly, since everyone is unique, how and to what extent side effects impact on you and your life needs to be taken into account by your healthcare providers. Side effects may not always be avoidable, but they can usually be reduced and managed. Unvoiced concerns about effectiveness or side effects and forgetfulness are all common reasons for not taking medication, for non-adherence, but they may also be addressed by discussing them with the team at the pharmacy.

ENTITLEMENTS

The cost of medications in Ireland is governed by an agreement between the pharmaceutical companies and the government. Medications are available through several schemes administered by the HSE. The price of your medications and the eligibility criteria for the different schemes will continue to vary over time as government policy and HSE regulations frequently change. Both your pharmacist and the HSE can help you determine what your entitlements are and how you should access whatever support is available.

PROVIDING AND ADVISING ABOUT THE USE OF NON-PRESCRIPTION MEDICINES AND SUPPLEMENTS

Non-prescription medications

Paracetamol and aspirin are available in non-pharmacy outlets as single ingredient analgesic preparations for pain relief, and together with ibuprofen they are available from pharmacies in both single ingredient and combination preparations. Combination preparations come in many types: two analgesics together – aspirin and paraceta-mol; one or two analgesics plus codeine; one or two analgesics plus caffeine – this may be included since it increases the effectiveness of aspirin and paracetamol (see below); and/or an anti-nauseant (also known as antiemetic) or a muscle relaxant may also be present.

It is important to check all of the ingredients because many sources of advice concentrate only on the analgesics and whether codeine is present or not and many healthcare professionals are unsure of the exact composition. This is not the full picture; the pack, the leaflet and one of the pharmacy team can help you because each of the ingredients has its advantages and disadvantages, and it is worth remembering that a particular combination may be useful in one circumstance and intolerable in another.

Paracetamol

Paracetamol at a dose of 1,000 mg is effective, well tolerated and easy to take, but the maximum daily dose for an adult is 4,000 mg or 4 g. Paracetamol may be less effective if a person delays taking it during the first symptoms of the migraine because the stomach slows down moving its contents into the intestines, which is where paracetamol is absorbed. Aspirin is used much less nowadays. Although it was effective in clinical trials, the dose used in those trials was higher than the authorised dose for non-prescription preparations (single dose 300–650 mg up to six times per day) and it is likely to produce upset stomach (gastrointestinal irritation), particularly in older people. It should be used for the minimum period possible, as the irritation may lead to more serious complications.

Ibuprofen

Ibuprofen is effective at a dose of 400 mg and is less likely to cause gastrointestinal upset, but no more than 1,200 mg should be used in one day and in older people it should be used for the minimum period possible. However, if you have experienced a skin rash soon after taking aspirin or ibuprofen, or if you notice that you are short of breath or feel chest tightness when breathing, you should switch to paracetamol and make an appointment to see your General Practitioner, because this sensitivity can lead to serious breathing difficulties. If you have any history of gastric or peptic ulceration, you should consult your General Practitioner or pharmacist before using either aspirin or ibuprofen.

Codeine

Codeine is only available without prescription in a number of countries around the world; this is indicative of the caution required when using it.

Codeine, while effective, is present in low doses in non-prescription preparations, and this can limit its effectiveness in a severe migraine attack. Unfortunately, constipation, which is a common side effect of codeine, occurs whatever dose is taken. Other effects, such as sedation and cognitive slowing (a decline in memory and thinking skills) in older people occur at the maximum recommended dose. Codeine-containing preparations are capable of inducing dependence if used continuously, and of giving rise to withdrawal symptoms when the codeine is stopped (see Medication Overuse Headache in earlier chapter). Pharmacy staff are well positioned to potentially identify possible customers at risk and provide further information and support on this.

Single ingredient analgesic preparations may be just as effective in mild to moderate migraine episodes as codeine-containing combinations and therefore they are not considered first-line preparations. To help promote the use of more appropriate treatment and to reduce the frequency of adverse effects and of misuse, codeine-containing preparations are kept in the dispensary and must be requested by patients.

Pharmacists are required to check with each patient to confirm the need and suitability of the preparation for the patient's condition.

Once again, this is a precaution that is consistent with the pharmacist's role in ensuring the responsible use of medications for society as a whole and should not be seen as a barrier to appropriate use by a patient in need. Non-prescription analgesics, which are the regular painkillers that can be bought over the counter, are required to carry advice on the pack that they should not be taken for more than three days without an assessment of the patient's condition.

Caffeine
Caffeine is frequently overlooked as an ingredient of analgesic preparations. Many paracetamol and paracetamol–codeine combination preparations contain caffeine in amounts ranging from 15–65 mg. While caffeine enhances the analgesic effect of paracetamol it also, as most people know, can keep us awake and can irritate the stomach; consequently caffeine may not allow the person experiencing migraine the chance to rest and, by irritating the stomach, may make feelings of nausea worse. Moreover, if used excessively on a daily basis, it can produce withdrawal symptoms when it is stopped. Whether these symptoms are worse when codeine is present in the preparation is not known, but prudence would suggest continuous use of both of these ingredients at maximum dosage is inadvisable.

Anti-nauseant drugs
Anti-nauseant drugs may be useful at the outset of a migraine attack but are of less value if taken later in an attack; that is why products such as Migraleve and motilium (domperidone) come in different formulations for these phases. Dry mouth and cognitive slowing, mainly in older people, are side effects that some people will experience.

Sensitivity to the effects of any ingredient in a medication is specific to an individual, so once you have determined how you respond, you should inform any healthcare provider who prescribes or recommends a product for your migraine and you should make sure they check out with you all the ingredients of any preparation that you have not used before; both the pack and the patient information leaflet carry a full list. All medications should only be used at the recommended dose and for the recommended duration – you should discuss your use of medication with your pharmacist or General Practitioner if you have specific questions.

Supplements and other preparations
Many different supplements, herbal preparations and other products are promoted as aids in preventing or treating migraine. However, in several cases the objective supporting evidence is poor; so, while the products are available and some people may feel they get benefit from them, pharmacists will not recommend them.

Riboflavin, Magnesium, Co-enzyme Q10 and *Pestasites hybridus* have shown some evidence of effectiveness to be regarded as credible preparations, but how they work is not known and, as with any drug when you first take it, you should monitor your response to see that it works for you and that there are no unusual effects.

Riboflavin is vitamin B2 and at 200 mg twice daily may prevent migraine. One unavoidable side effect is that as the drug and its breakdown products appear in the urine, they make it intensely yellow or even orange. This is nothing to worry about and any stains on underwear will wash out.

Co-enzyme Q10 also occurs in the body and acts rather like a vitamin to assist in the metabolic processes (chemical reactions) of most cells. It is known for its antioxidant activity (which counters damaging effects on cells). At a dose of up to 300 mg per day it can reduce the frequency of migraine episodes with the possibility of gastrointestinal upset.

Magnesium oxide (400–600 mg) may be of benefit in preventing migraine, but the evidence is not clear-cut and diarrhoea is a potential side effect.

ASSESSING AND ADVISING PATIENTS ABOUT SYMPTOMS

Because headaches are common and everyone has some experience of them, everyone feels that they can tell one type from another. Nevertheless, when headaches are unusually severe, frequent or prolonged, show a different pattern of symptoms or are made worse by something that previously was innocuous, or are not relieved by a medication that was effective before, then this needs to be assessed – and pharmacists are usually trained to do this. You will have to spend some time giving your pharmacist a full history of your symptoms and your other medical history. If the pharmacist considers that you need to see a General Practitioner or recommends that you see your Neurologist, they will tell you. Pharmacists often refer people in this way and it is important to act upon their advice when, in their professional judgement, a more detailed and comprehensive assessment of your symptoms is needed.

OTHER NON-PHARMACOLOGICAL MEASURES

There are many non-pharmacological steps that can be taken to reduce the frequency and severity of migraine. Advice from the Migraine Association, combined with your own experience of what makes it better and what makes it worse, will be the most productive approach. Other non-pharmacological or non-drug options available in pharmacies include:

Migrastick

The Migrastick is a roller-ball stick of peppermint and lavender essential oils in a small tube which can be carried around in a purse or pocket. It has a cooling effect when applied to the temples, forehead and nape of the neck at the first sign of headache. Each stick contains about 100 applications. It is available in most pharmacies and health food stores, but it is not suitable for use when pregnant or breastfeeding.

The Migra-Cap

The Migra-Cap was developed by a migraine sufferer. It combines cold therapy with complete darkness to give relief from the pain associated with migraine and most types of headache. It is suitable for every member of the family and can be stored in an ordinary domestic fridge or freezer until needed. The Migra-Cap is available from McCabe's or McDaid's pharmacies.

The Paingone Pen

The Paingone Pen is a plastic pen-like device that generates an electronic pulse to stimulate the release of endorphins (natural pain-fighters) into the bloodstream. It is based on Transcutaneous (through the skin) Nerve Stimulation (TNS), uses an electrical current to stimulate nerves and can be applied immediately to the area of pain. It should not be used by people with epilepsy, pregnant women or people fitted with a pacemaker. Use of the Paingone Pen by children under eight years of age should be supervised. The device is available in some pharmacies.

USE OF THE INTERNET TO PURCHASE MEDICATION

For medication or supplement or other forms of treatment you should only purchase products from reputable manufacturers and suppliers. Just because it is cheap and advertised on the Internet does not make it a good bargain, and in some instances it may be dangerous. Medications without any active ingredient, or with undeclared active ingredients are frequently promoted via Internet sites claiming to be pharmacies, and every year in Ireland a number of people are admitted to hospital because of falsified medicines obtained from unregulated and unauthorised sources. If you are in any doubt, look at the Pharmacy Regulator site (www.thepsi.ie) and the Healthcare Products Regulatory Authority website (www.hpra.ie) for information and advice about Internet Pharmacies.

Research in Ireland and other countries has shown that unless a Medication Use Review is performed by a pharmacist with all of the relevant information, serious medication-related problems may occur that directly put the patient's health at risk. Pharmacists' recommendations may take many forms, not only suggesting additional medications if needed, but also discontinuation of medications that are no longer required. A pharmacist will always be willing to hear about medication from a patient and to pass on that information on behalf of the patient to other healthcare providers if the patient wishes.

Effectively and responsibly used, medication can be a great boon to patients. Migraine can be controlled and its impact minimised if patients make the most of their pharmacy and their pharmacist.

5

HEADACHES IN GENERAL PRACTICE
& WOMEN AND MIGRAINE

Dr Paddy Daly

Dr Paddy Daly qualified in medicine through UCD and St Vincent's Hospital. He was one of three to found a group practice in Dun Laoghaire which grew into a large teaching practice, allowing the development of special skills and services. Migraine was one of these, which in more recent years led him to practice in the migraine clinic at St Vincent's.

Over the years Paddy attended many of the major headache conferences in the world and for six years was a Board member of the Migraine Association of Ireland. He has run several headache training events accredited by the Irish College of GPs.

INTRODUCTION

Headaches are a common problem seen in general practice, ranging in their severity and disability and occasionally having an underlying serious cause. In Ireland it is estimated about 13,000 people suffer from migraine alone on a daily basis, with all the misery and loss of opportunity that accompany the disorder.

There are many other causes of headache, all of which need accurate diagnosis and treatment plans for the best outcomes. We are lucky in Ireland to have a well-developed specialty of general practice.

Not only do General Practitioners (GPs) have postgraduate degrees in their specialty, but they are well distributed throughout the country.

Access to a general practitioner – except, perhaps, in some rural areas – is not a problem and usually it is possible to see a GP on the day requested. GPs also work with their patients under the distinct advantage that the GP is normally chosen by the patient. This implies that a good relationship exists which enables care for all age groups and enhances outcomes. Many headache conditions are chronic (persistent over time and occurring on fifteen days or more per month) and require ongoing care. Most GPs work within mixed professional groups and so they can call on other professional expertise, such as physiotherapy, as required.

Migraine, in particular, affects women far more than men, and the explanation for this lies in the varying hormonal cycle. Interventions in this cycle to improve migraine is something GPs are especially well equipped to do.

DIAGNOSIS

Research in Ireland reveals the uncomfortable fact that it takes, on average, seven years for someone to get an accurate diagnosis for their headache. This implies that the person has had inadequate treatment for a long time and is still looking for help. Further, the person has probably been self-medicating during this time and exposing themselves to the misuse of such tablets.

Getting a firm diagnosis for your headache is therefore important and your GP should be well able to help you achieve that. There is, perhaps, one situation where it is best to go to an Emergency Department. That is where you undergo a sudden, unexpected and previously unexperienced very severe headache. This is often called a 'thunderclap headache', which describes it very well. It may represent a bleed from an artery within the head and requires urgent specialised care.

The headaches which a GP sees most often include migraine, tension headache, medication overuse headache and headache from neck problems. Occasionally, he/she will see someone with cluster headache, headache associated with obesity called idiopathic intracranial hypertension, and headaches as part of other diseases.

Reaching a correct diagnosis takes time. During your visit, the GP will want to take a detailed history, examine you, take into account other medical conditions you may have, consider investigations and finally put all that together into a personalised treatment plan for you.

PLANNING YOUR VISIT

o Ask the secretary if longer than average visits are available.
o Try not to visit accompanied by children. They get bored and, if upset, cause distraction. There is a lot of detail to get from you in the history. Further, there may be a lot of new information coming to you which you will need to remember.
o It is a good idea to bring someone with you who knows you well and whom you trust. Others see us differently to how we see ourselves. For example, it is of interest to know how you feel before your migraine headache begins. You may not be aware of any change in you, but a partner might well volunteer that your mood does change, and they will know you are heading towards a migraine before you do! Knowing this allows for more precise treatment.
o Enduring a chronic illness may lead to tolerance of some symptoms which you then forget to mention. Hearing the comments about you and how the headaches affect you and your relationships is important to know. Indeed, the person accompanying you may well benefit from venting their concerns and knowing that a full assessment is underway.

At a first visit, your doctor will want to carry out a physical examination of the nervous system. This will not be intrusive and will be expected to be normal for migraine, tension headaches, and cluster headache. While not wanting to repeat what is explained in the chapter on triggers for migraine, I might mention one trigger which, as a GP, I would have commonly seen – and that is the issue of neck problems.

It is surprising how many migraine sufferers show some problem in their necks. Whatever the cause, maybe poor posture or old injury, it will be essential to have your neck checked by a chartered physiotherapist and appropriate treatment commenced if any neck issues are found.

The diagnosis may include consideration of other medical conditions which may aggravate migraine, such as diabetes or thyroid problems. The doctor will also want to weigh you if you appear to be overweight. Obesity is a serious threat to changing migraine from an occasional attack to occurring frequently and becoming chronic. By definition migraine is said to be chronic when occurring on fifteen days or more per month. Being obese changes risk of this happening from 1 in 32 for slim people to 1 in 6 when obese.

Obesity itself may lead to a particular type of headache called idiopathic intracranial hypertension. This idiopathic (cause uncertain or unknown) intracranial (inside the skull) hyptertension (abnormally high pressure) particularly affects obese women in their twenties. Given the large rise in the numbers of overweight people it is likely to be seen more often and will be picked up by your GP during the examination.

Establishing the diagnosis of migraine may, therefore, lead to some subsidiary diagnoses. As stated, many people do not get a diagnosis for years. This may be because of infrequent attacks which resolve quickly, but some caution is needed if your migraine is increasing in frequency, or if you get clear-cut migraines interspersed with more vague, tension-type headaches.

This is often the scenario where excess use of pain tablets begins. Pain tablet use on more than ten days per month is defined as medication overuse and may lead into more headache days. The diagnosis at that point moves from migraine to 'medication overuse headache' also. If you recognise any of this, then please attend to it early as treatment becomes more difficult the longer it is delayed. Pain tablets should be used on no more than four days per month.

CHILDREN

Children also get headaches and are likely to be brought to the GP first. Migraine is hereditary and the expression of the genes may occur at an early age. Migraine in children may not be as clearly defined as in adults, and headaches should not be assumed to be migraine even where there is a family history of migraine. As stated above, a consultation under calm conditions applies equally for children.

Much of the history will come from the parent, but most children can communicate well by six or seven years of age and should be allowed to do so with the GP. The child will probably know the GP anyway, which will be helpful. Do not be surprised if the GP takes a broad view of the problem. Stress is the most common trigger for migraine. In children this will require exploration of issues such as bullying, or stress arising at home from siblings, or discord between parents if they are going through a difficult time. The possibility of abuse is always considered now in any situation where a child is stressed. Children can find it very difficult to vocalise concerns in these areas, so the GP may use the consultation to raise your awareness as a parent.

A further thought in the GP's mind when examining a child will be whether a sinister cause could account for the headaches. While rare, brain tumours in children do occur and will be considered. This raises the question of whether adults and children should have brain scans routinely to aid the diagnosis of migraine. Where the history is clearly one of migraine over a period of time and the physical examination is normal it is not essential in adults to order an MRI brain scan. Many, of course, would ask for such for reassurance, which is perfectly understandable, and the GP can easily arrange for this to be done privately. However, GPs do not have access to such scans in the public hospitals and would have to refer to the outpatients first. Long delays are to be expected. For children, the need for scanning is clearer. As children they may not have been around long enough for the cyclic nature of migraine to be obvious, their migraine may be less developed and recognisable and the chances of something else being the cause of their headache is higher. A decision to refer will need to be discussed with the parent.

MIGRAINE AND WOMEN

While young boys and girls are equally subject to migraine, this begins to change as they go through puberty. Many boys stop having migraine, but the frequency increases in girls. Often it is in the teen years that migraine first manifests itself. Ultimately, migraine becomes about three times more common in women than in men. The incidence continues to increase throughout early adult life, reaches a peak at about forty years of age, and then slowly declines. This variation is due to hormonal reasons. In boys the hormone levels are steady, but they are variable in girls.

In women the migraine pattern may follow two courses. Firstly, the attacks may remain random and have no regular association with the menstrual cycle. For others the attacks may be wholly confined to the onset of menstruation and rarely occur at other times. Usually there is an individual pattern for each woman which repeats itself in a reliable way. Thus, the attack for some might start on day one of the period and for others earlier or later. Menstruation is the end of the cycle and results from not being pregnant. Over the preceding two weeks the body has been preparing for pregnancy with a rise in hormones. These hormone levels then drop, precipitating the period and triggering migraine. In rare cases, a woman may be sensitive to the small drop in hormones that occurs mid-cycle prior to ovulation. Menstrual migraine is rarely accompanied by visual aura.

Menstrual migraine is treated with the usual available medications but can be more difficult to reduce. However, it is open to hormonal manipulation using medications with which your GP is very familiar. Treatment plans will still require a review of other triggers, as a woman may be more sensitive to them with the hormonal drop.

If the cycle is regular, then the day the migraine attack is due can be calculated and a mini prophylaxis (preventative) plan used. Use of a Triptan agent such as Frovex taken the night before can work well. Other Triptans can be tried but the longer working ones such as Frovex and Nariverg are usually best. These may be used with an anti-inflammatory agent as well, such as Nurofen, aspirin or a prescription item. The latter are also useful for reducing menstrual pain and if that is a problem then it is a good idea to take the anti-inflammatory regularly for three days before the period is due. Knowing the number of days the migraine usually lasts determines the number of nights the Triptan and anti-inflammatory are taken.

Another approach is to suppress the cycle by use of a depot progesterone injection such as Depo-Provera, which is given at twelve-weekly intervals. Implanon, progesterone in the form of a rod implanted under the skin in the upper arm, may also be helpful. The Mirena coil also contains progesterone and does prevent menstrual migraine for some women. Oral versions of progesterone contraception such as Noriday and Cerazette do not suppress the ovulation cycle sufficiently to prevent menstrual migraine.

There is yet another variation to consider. As stated, menstrual migraine is precipitated by the drop in oestrogen levels in the days leading up to the period. Oestrogen supplementation during these days reduces the drop and may be enough to prevent the onset of migraine. Some women find it only postpones the attack and, in such situations, the supplementation may need to be maintained for a week until natural oestrogen levels are rising again. The oestrogen is usually given in the form of a gel which is rubbed onto the skin daily for the duration required. Divigel is one such product commonly available.

All of the above medications are regularly used by women as a means of contraception and for much of the time may neatly fill two roles. All GPs work with women and their contraceptive needs on a daily basis and are highly experienced at advising on their suitability for the individual woman.

Another approach to the problem is to suppress the menstrual cycle entirely. This can be achieved by use of the combined oral contraceptive pill continuously without a break from one packet to the next. It is acceptable practice to continue this for six months before taking a week's break and then continuing for another six months. In this way migraine attacks may be reduced to only two per year.

There is one exception to the information above. About 20% of women experience visual aura with migraine, and in those circumstances the use of the combined oral contraceptive pill is not advised. This is because such women have an increased risk of stroke with that type of migraine. The risk is very small but has been established as a fact. Using the combined pill as a contraceptive increases that small risk and, therefore, is contraindicated. However, all the progesterone-only products available are entirely safe to use for women who have migraine with aura. The risk is related to the frequency of migraine: the more frequent the migraine, the greater is the risk. If migraine is occurring several times a month then preventative medication could be considered rather than relying on repeated acute treatments. It is important for such women to be mindful of their general health and not inadvertently increase their risk by smoking or by becoming overweight.

Pregnancy for the woman with migraine requires some forward planning. Fortunately, pregnancy brings an improvement in migraine for most women due to the rising hormone levels and so there is less need for medications. This is just as well, as the initial starting point for advice is that all the acute treatments you may be using are undesirable, at best, during pregnancy. Many women have used Triptan drugs in the early weeks before they realise they are pregnant and there have been no foetal problems identified. Nevertheless, you should stop using them when pregnant, as they may influence blood flow to the uterus. All anti-inflammatory drugs are undesirable as they increase the risk of miscarriage. Your GP or pharmacist will help you identify the nature of tablets you are unsure of. In pregnancy all herbal remedies should be seen as unreliable products as to what they contain and should be avoided.

There is another range of medications used for migraine prevention that ideally, if you are taking them, you should discuss plans for pregnancy well ahead of allowing a pregnancy to occur. The most common groups of drugs you may be on include what are called beta blockers, tricyclic anti-depressants, anti-epileptic drugs and others more commonly used in cardiac conditions. It is particularly important that you should not be on the epileptic treatments such as Topamax or Epilim during pregnancy. They cause serious foetal abnormalities and almost universally cause childhood developmental problems. It has become best practice in clinics to ask a woman to sign a consent document prior to initiating such drugs to make sure that she understands the risks.

The only preventative medication in which there is any room for use is with beta blockers. There is no risk of foetal abnormality, but the growth of the baby would need close observation by the obstetrician. Close co-operation is the key. If migraine is difficult during pregnancy there are a few safe ways to provide help, but these would usually only be available though special migraine clinics. Procedures such as nerve blocks and use of nerve stimulators are available and some GPs have trained in their use.

Once the baby is born, you will need to discuss with your GP when you can safely return to your preventative medications. If you are breastfeeding some are not allowed as they are excreted in the milk. Anti-inflammatory drugs such as Nurofen and beta blockers are compatible, but there would be concerns with the anti-epileptic and anti-depressant drugs. Occipital nerve blocks, as in pregnancy, are allowed. Of the Triptan drugs, Imigran (sumatriptan) is compatible with breastfeeding and is best taken immediately after the baby has been fed. The use of the other Triptans is uncertain.

Breastfeeding is not associated with the exacerbation of migraine. General care such as good hydration, support and relaxation techniques will all play a role in allowing you and your baby to thrive. This is a time of profound change for all women, but particularly so after a first baby. Coming to terms with all the implications for life and living can become overwhelming for some people, especially with migraine thrown in as well. Your GP is there to help address your worries and rationalise the medical treatments required.

6

HEADACHE/MIGRAINE CLINICS
& MIGRAINE IN SPORT

Dr Edward M. O'Sullivan

Dr Edward O'Sullivan has a GP Practice in Bishopstown in Cork. He has been Clinical Director of the Cork University Migraine Clinic since its foundation in 2000 and has a long-term interest in headache disorders. He recently published a research paper on migraine headache presentations in pharmacies which was accepted for the International Headache Society Annual Congress in Boston and published in the Irish Medical Journal. He is Medical Advisor to the Migraine Association of Ireland.

INTRODUCTION

Headache is a common complaint and within the community there is a lifetime prevalence of over 90% and a yearly prevalence of 40%. In other words, more than 90% of people will experience headache in their lifetime and on a yearly basis 40% of people will suffer headache. The peak prevalence occurs in middle age. Most of these headache sufferers are routinely and effectively managed in primary care. Nevertheless, for many, headaches go undiagnosed, are wrongly diagnosed or are difficult to diagnose correctly.

Headache disorders are frequently associated with high levels of disability, reduced productivity, and impact greatly on the individual, their families and the workplace. The findings, in a large European

MIGRAINE

study in women with migraine aged between 18–35 years, found that they lost two days from work and had four additional days of functional disability at work or home in the previous six months. They also highlighted that their migraine affected their career ambitions, promotion and participation in leisure activities.

For many individuals the commonly used over-the-counter analgesics or painkillers and standard therapies are often only of limited benefit, and their headaches progress to control and dominate many aspects of their lives. The resulting disability means that these patients suffer in silence and have many unmet needs.

Patient support groups have highlighted their plight and the Migraine Association of Ireland has been to the forefront in raising awareness. The Association has successfully lobbied on their behalf: the medical profession, the HSE (health service executive), politicians, governments and others. It actively promotes greater awareness, investment, education, research and a prioritisation of their healthcare needs.

It is against this background that the need for specialist Headache/Migraine clinics emerged. The first dedicated headache clinic dates back to the 1930s in the Massachusetts General Hospital. However, it has only been in recent decades that specialist Headache/Migraine clinics have numerically increased in great numbers both across the United States and Europe. These clinics are dedicated to the management of benign (i.e. not malignant) headache disorders and are recognised as an important resource in the care of those who suffer from debilitating refractory headaches (headaches that are resistant to treatment), particularly migraine.

In Ireland there are five Headache/Migraine clinics; all operate within neurology departments and are affiliated to teaching hospitals. Headache/Migraine clinics are made up of multidisciplinary teams and adopt an integrated headache programme in the care of patients. The team is led by either a clinical neurologist or a doctor with a special interest and expertise in headache management. The team members include trainee neurology registrars, other trainee doctors, clinical nurse specialists, physiotherapists, psychologists, cognitive behavioural therapists and occupational therapists.

In addition, timely access to diagnostics, particularly radiological neuroimaging, is an essential component in the delivery of headache services. Consultation at the clinics is by appointment and referrals may come from many sources, including General Practitioners, neurologists, neurosurgeons, emergency departments, ear nose and throat surgeons, other physicians, psychiatrists, physiotherapists and opticians. Headache/Migraine clinics are considered tertiary referral centres, as many patients have already consulted a number of doctors and other healthcare professionals prior to their outpatient attendance.

Headache/Migraine clinics at their best make significant contributions in three key areas:

1. Clinical evaluation and patient care.
2. Medical education.
3. Research.

CLINICAL EVALUATION AND PATIENT CARE

The management of headache patients is the primary function of a specialist Headache/Migraine service. Clinical evaluation recognises that whilst headache is the presenting symptom (the main complaint or reason given for seeking treatment), the use of the term migraine requires a diagnosis based on an accurate, detailed history and examination. The indications for referral to the clinic range from:

o When there is confusion or doubt about the diagnosis.
o Patients who are unresponsive or poorly responsive to either acute and/or preventative therapies.
o Patients with Chronic Daily Headache, particularly Chronic Migraine.
o Patients with Chronic Daily Headache and Medication Overuse Headache.

o New Daily Persistent Headache.
o Patients with co-morbid (the greater then co-incidental existence of two conditions occurring in the same condition) psychiatric and anxiety states.
o Patients with other severe, albeit rare, debilitating headache disorders such as: cluster headache, chronic paroxysmal hemicranias, post-traumatic headaches and short-lasting stabbing headaches.

In many Headache/Migraine clinics, prior to their consultation, patients are asked to complete questionnaires and to keep headache diaries. These diaries chronicle the frequency, duration, headache characteristics, associated symptoms, trigger factors, impact and the effectiveness of their therapies. This preparation yields valuable clinical details and helps to maximise the consultation between the headache specialist and the patient at the first attendance. The demographic features (statistical features of a section of the population) of clinic patients repeatedly show a mean age of forty years and a female: male ratio of 2.5:1.

HISTORY TAKING

The first responsibility of a headache specialist is to make a clinical diagnosis based on a comprehensive history and examination. Worldwide, in the modern era, most clinicians incorporate and use the International Headache Society's classification of headache disorders guidelines (ICHD, 3rd edition) as a useful diagnostic tool. This provides for standardisation of care and conformity of medical opinion. It enables clinical data from differing ethnic, cultural and social backgrounds to be compared across the globe.

Secondary causes for headaches such as brain tumours and cerebral (brain) aneurysms (excessive swelling of the wall of an artery), although rare, are an important consideration in the differential diagnosis and their potential cause leads to anxiety for many patients. Therefore timely access, when indicated, to brain imaging (CT Scan and MRI) along with laboratory blood tests is routinely available in the initial care plan.

The first consultation with the headache specialist is comprehensive, lengthy and detailed. The history taking outlines:

1. The number of years and age of onset of first headache; the frequency and duration of attacks.
2. The doctor explores in great detail any preceding aura or premonitory symptoms (warning signs) prior to the headache.
3. The characteristics of the headache, the severity, the presence of associated symptoms and the impact and disability caused by attacks.
4. The specialist reviews all treatments that the patient has tried to date, including acute and preventive therapies and non-drug therapies.
5. The specialist evaluates how effective patients are at self-medicating with over-the-counter analgesics (e.g. paracetamol or ibuprofen or aspirin).
6. Have they ever been prescribed specific migraine therapies (e.g. Triptans) and how effective were these?
7. Have they ever been prescribed preventative therapies (e.g. propranolol, topiramate), how long have they continuously taken them for (weeks, months or years) and how useful were they in reducing the frequency, severity and duration of their headaches?
8. Have they ever used non-drug therapies such as relaxation therapies, physiotherapy, acupuncture or psychological counselling?
9. Does the patient have any co-existing co-morbid (existing at the same time) medical conditions such as depression or anxiety states?

At the end of the consultation the headache specialist will be in a position to make a definitive diagnosis.

Numerous studies and audits in peer-reviewed journals repeatedly demonstrate that episodic and chronic migraine with or without medication overuse are the most frequently diagnosed headache disorders at the clinics. Cluster headache, although a rare condition compared to migraine, is also commonly encountered at the clinics.

In contrast, even though Tension-Type Headache is the most common headache disorder in the community, it is seldom seen in Headache/Migraine clinics. This reflects their usual mild, self-limiting nature and associated low levels of disability. Tension-Type Headaches are in general easy to manage with simple analgesics (e.g. paracetamol or aspirin) and patients seldom need to consult their general practitioners or seek professional advice.

A detailed list of the likely headache disorders diagnosed at clinics is listed below.

o Episodic Migraine With and Without Aura.
o Chronic Migraine (> 15 days per month).
o Chronic Migraine + Medication Overuse.
o New Daily Persistent Headache.
o Episodic Cluster Headache.
o Chronic Cluster Headache.
o Post-Traumatic Headaches.
o Cervicogenic Headaches (caused by neck disorder or lesion).
o Chronic Tension-Type Headache.
o Other benign causes of headache.
o Other rare secondary causes (e.g. brain tumour, Arnold-Chiari malformation; cerebral aneurysms are rare < 1%).

After making the diagnosis, it is the priority of the headache specialist to formulate a treatment plan which co-ordinates the management options and monitors their progress. Patients are given a clear explanation of their diagnosis and the underlying pathophysiological mechanisms of their headache disorder. Specific acute and preventative therapies are prescribed, where indicated, and these recommendations will need to be closely monitored and evaluated at subsequent follow-up appointments. In addition, at the clinics, specific preventative treatment options such as occipital nerve blockade and subcutaneous Botulinum Toxin A (Botox) injections are provided for suitably identified patients.

To monitor progress between outpatient appointments, all patients are given a headache diary and asked to keep an accurate account outlining in detail their future attacks. Data recorded within the headache diaries includes:

o The frequency, duration and severity of attack.

o The presence or otherwise of trigger factors which are identifiable in 20–30% of patients, the most frequent being different forms of personal or work-related stress and lifestyle situations such as lack of sleep, over-tiredness and missed meals. Other triggers include the menstrual cycle, dietary factors and alcohol.

o The clinical features of the headaches outlining the location, character and severity.

o The presence or absence of other symptoms (e.g. nausea/vomiting, intolerance to light and or sound).

o The impact of attacks utilising disability questionnaires such as MIDAS (Migraine Disability Assessment) and HIT (Headache Impact Test) tests.

o The effectiveness of acute therapies and particularly the time it takes to provide meaningful pain relief, which ideally is in less than two hours.

o The effectiveness of any preventative therapy in reducing the frequency, severity and duration of attacks. Preventative therapies can also enhance the effectiveness of their acute therapies.

The headache specialist will also identify those patients who would potentially benefit from a referral to a member of the multidisciplinary team. It is recognised that pharmacotherapy (medication) on its own will only improve the outcome and reduce the number of headache days for approximately 50% of patients with debilitating headache disorders such as chronic migraine and Medication Overuse Headache.

THE ROLE OF THE NURSE

Clinical nurse specialists have evolved in recent years across many specialties and are an integral part of Headache/Migraine Clinics. They work closely with the headache specialist and other team members in key clinical areas. They are a valuable resource in providing:

o Additional consultation time with patients who require further explanation of their diagnosis.
o Education on all aspects of their care.
o Advice on acute and preventative therapies and their side effects.
o The need for compliance and adherence to their treatment recommendations.
o Explanations on the reasoning behind medication changes and potential benefits of these changes.
o Advice on trigger factors and their avoidance.
o The nurse specialist, who can make further treatment changes and recommendations, reviews many patients at their follow-up clinical appointment. The nurse, where necessary, will liaise with the headache specialist when there are any challenging management decisions to be discussed. In this way the workload at clinics can be maximised.
o Between clinic appointments the nurse is a vital link person and provides telephone advice to patients. This is an important function as there are often many months between appointments.

PHYSIOTHERAPY

Those patients whose headaches are accompanied by musculoskeletal neck pain/stiffness are frequently referred to the physiotherapist, who will do their own history and examination and recommend a specifically designed treatment programme. The goal of physiotherapy is primarily prevention and to reduce the frequency of attacks. Patients frequently require a number of treatment sessions before a benefit is seen. Cervicogenic headache, post-traumatic headaches and migraine patients with accompanying neck stiffness do best from a referral to the physiotherapist (see Chapter 8).

PSYCHIATRIC EVALUATION AND PSYCHOLOGICAL COUNSELLING

30–50% of the workload at Headache/Migraine clinics is made up of Chronic Daily Headache (> 15 days per month) and Medication Overuse Headache (MOH). Many of these patients have co-morbid depression and anxiety states. These patient groups are the least likely to do well with pharmacotherapy on its own. Therefore, many are referred to the psychiatric and psychological services that will carefully access for an underlying co-morbid depression/anxiety illness and the presence of psychosocial stressors.

A depressive illness is treated in its own right by the psychiatric team and effective management of the underlying depression can also lead to an improvement in the headaches.

Stress is commonly regarded as an important trigger in both episodic and chronic migraine. Stress manifests itself in many forms ranging from personal, work-related or financial to lifestyle (over-tiredness, lack of sleep), all of which have an impact and lower the individual's headache threshold. Management options include: cognitive behavioural therapy, counselling, stress management, relaxation therapies, exercise, lifestyle interventions and better personal time management. These interventions combined with their medications are known to improve the outcome for many patients.

EDUCATION

Specialist Headache/Migraine clinics play a central role in the area of headache education. Key areas of education are:

o Education of the patient: In management plans, educating the patient about their symptoms, diagnosis and treatments is routine.

It is considered one of the most important functions of the clinics and is aided by patient information leaflets produced by the Migraine Association of Ireland. Educated, informed patients achieve a better clinical outcome and many studies have repeatedly demonstrated this.

o Education of Medical Trainees: Doctors in training, particularly neurological and general practice trainees, get valuable clinical exposure and experience by doing a rotation through a headache clinic. This gives rise to a new generation of medical practitioners in both primary and secondary care whose knowledge and understanding of headache management will enhance the lives of many headache and migraine sufferers into the future.

o Undergraduate Teaching: In Ireland, the Headache/Migraine clinics are divisions within neurology departments and have close links with the universities and teaching hospitals. These affiliations enable headache disorders to be part of the undergraduate teaching programme for medical students and others including pharmacy students. This programme includes didactic lectures, small group meetings and student attachments. Medical students also get to attend the clinics and observe experienced headache specialists taking histories and examinations. This undergraduate programme ensures that medical students get the opportunity to learn about the importance of headache disorders and their accompanying disability early on in their careers.

RESEARCH

Academic research undertaken at specialist Headache/Migraine clinics is a valuable resource in furthering our understanding and knowledge of headache disorders. Research, in addition, raises the profile amongst the general public and facilitates the many awareness campaigns highlighting the plight of those disabled by headache.

The study of this patient cohort yields important information in the key clinical areas of:

o The diagnosis and spectrum of headache disorders referred to clinics.

o The epidemiology and demographics (age and sex, socio-economic factors) of those attending clinics.

o The level of disability caused by severe headache disorders, particularly migraine, using validated questionnaires such as the MIDAS and HIT tests.

o The efficacy and benefits of treatments (acute, preventative, physiotherapy and other non-drug therapies) of those attending clinics.

o Published research. The clinic database enables numerous specific areas of headache medicine to be studied and published in peer-reviewed journals. In particular, little was known about Medication Overuse Headache until recent times. Much of our current knowledge and ongoing research has been undertaken at specialist Headache/Migraine clinics.

o Clinical drug trials. Worldwide, many phase 2 and late phase 3 drug trials are undertaken at Headache/Migraine clinics. New medications, focusing on providing relief from the acute attack and the prevention of future attacks are the driving force behind research. Research strives towards addressing the disability and unmet needs of those disabled by episodic migraine, chronic migraine, Medication Overuse Headache and other benign headache disorders.

CONCLUSIONS

Specialist Headache/Migraine clinics that either stand alone or, as in Ireland, within neurology departments, have been increasing in numbers in recent years across the world. It is recognised that specialisation enables a multidisciplinary approach to headache management, particularly for severe migraine, chronic migraine and Medication Overuse Headache. In numerous studies improved outcomes for those with refractory, disabling headache are best achieved by the care provided at Headache/Migraine clinics.

MIGRAINE IN SPORT

INTRODUCTION

Migraine is a common disorder in the community and the incidence increases rapidly between the ages of sixteen to thirty years. It has a peak prevalence in those in their thirties and forties. Exercise is a known potential trigger for migraine attacks and this has major implications for migraineurs engaged in leisure sports, competitive sports and high-performance athletics. In a study of migraineurs, 38% identified physical activity and sports as a trigger for at least some of their attacks. This resulted for many in the need to give up any offending sports.

Regular mild exercise, on the other hand, is often recommended for patients who experience frequent migraine attacks. The neuropeptide and endorphin release during this form of exercise can protect patients from future attacks, lower individual stress and improve mood.

MODERATE TO SEVERE EXERCISE AND SPORTS AS A TRIGGER

Physical exercise, either alone or in combination with other triggers, is a potential risk for individuals to reach their migraine threshold and precipitate a migraine attack. The combination of exercise with lifestyle triggers is particularly important; these include:

o Overtiredness.
o Lack of sleep.
o Missed meals.
o Stress.
o Dehydration.
o Change of routine.

MECHANISMS OF ACTION OF HEADACHE INDUCED BY SPORT

The underlying pathogenesis (origin and chain of development) of headache is better understood in recent years. It is thought to be due to activation of pain-sensitive fibres in the dura (hard outermost membrane covering the brain), central activation of pain fibres innervating the large intracranial blood vessels and meninges (membranes covering the brain), and dysfunction of central brainstem structures normally involved in pain processing.

MANAGEMENT OF EXERCISE-INDUCED MIGRAINE

General management advice and preparation prior to planned exercise and sports is important in limiting and preventing the onset of a migraine attack. These practical measures include:

o To be well rested prior to planned sporting activity.
o Eat within a few hours of the exercise, particularly foods containing slow-release carbohydrates.
o Stay well hydrated before, during and after the exercise.
o Rest following exercise.

The most effective acute therapies for the treatment of exercise-induced migraine are the specific anti-migraine therapies, the Triptans, which are serotonin 5HT1B/1D receptor antagonists. These agents are faster acting when given via nasal formulation and between 71–90% of footballers in the referenced study 5 got complete relief within two hours. The Triptans however are associated with side effect risks and these medications have the potential to narrow the coronary arteries. Therefore prior to their use underlying cardiac conditions need to be ruled out and patients should have an exercise ECG and an echocardiograph.

An alternative first-line acute treatment option is the combination of an anti-inflammatory non-steroidal analgesic such as ibuprofen with an anti-nausea agent such as domperidone. As with the treatment of all migraine attacks, acute therapies should be taken as early as possible after the onset of symptoms.

POST-TRAUMATIC MIGRAINE

Contact sports frequently result in either a direct or indirect head injury, which puts individuals at risk of developing post-traumatic headaches, the most debilitating of which is post-traumatic migraine. Head injury causes either a linear acceleration/deceleration or a rotational movement of the head and neck depending on the direction of forces on impact. There is poor correlation between the severity of the head injury and the risk of onset of headaches, and individuals are just as likely to suffer from headaches following a relatively minor head injury.

Post-traumatic headache is defined as the onset of headache within one week of the injury. It frequently begins within the first twenty-four hours and is often accompanied by concussive symptoms of:

o Poor memory.
o Poor concentration.
o Delayed reaction time.
o Change of mood/irritability.
o Sleep disturbance.

If the headache characteristics fulfil the diagnostic criteria for migraine they are then defined as post-traumatic migraine. Most patients' headaches spontaneously resolve over a period of weeks to a few months. When the migraine attacks persist beyond three months they are then defined as chronic post-traumatic migraine.

In many sports, particularly rugby, there is a mandatory period of rest following a concussive head injury. Treatment recommendations include the following:

o Symptomatic treatment of the headaches with simple analgesics (paracetamol, aspirin or ibuprofen) or Triptan therapies for migraine. Codeine-based products need to be avoided as they are banned substances by many sporting bodies and they also put the individual at risk of developing Medication Overuse Headache.
o Complete physical and psychological rest.
o Subsequent follow-up assessment and evaluation for symptomatic improvement.
o A gradual return to sporting activities following improvement.
o Consider the commencement of preventative therapies (e.g. amitriptyline 10 mg daily) for individuals whose headaches persist beyond 2–3 months and develop chronic post-traumatic migraine.

REFERENCES

o Clifford Rose, F., and Lipton, R.B., 'Headache clinics' (1993).
o Diener, H.C., et al., 'Integrated headache care', *Cephalalgia*, 31.9 (2011): 1039–1047.
o Pedraza, M.I., et al., 'Characteristics of the first 2000 patients registered in a specialist headache clinic', *Neurología (English Edition)*, 30.4 (2015): 208–213.
o Kernick, David P., and Goadsby, Peter J., 'Guidance for the management of headache in sport on behalf of The Royal College of General Practitioners and The British Association for the Study of Headache', *Cephalalgia*, 31.1 (2011): 106–111.
o McCrory, P., Heywood, J., and Ugoni, A., 'Open label study of intranasal sumatriptan (Imigran) for footballer's headache', *British journal of sports medicine*, 39.8 (2005): 552–554.

7

PHYSIOTHERAPY AND MIGRAINE

Julie Sugrue

Julie Sugrue is a Clinical Specialist Physiotherapist. She worked as part of the multidisciplinary team at Beaumont Hospital Headache Clinic for six years, before taking up her current post in the Pain Management Services. Julie qualified with a BSc (Hons) degree in Physiotherapy from the Royal College of Surgeons in Ireland (RCSI) in 2004, and completed her Master of Manual Therapy degree at the University or Western Australia, Perth, in 2007. This is where she developed an interest in the management of persistent pain conditions and headache, and proceeded to carry out more specific postgraduate training with international experts and neurology specialists in relation to headache.

INTRODUCTION

This chapter will focus on the role of physiotherapy in the management of migraine. Specifically the role of physiotherapy in the management of the neck pain associated with migraine. The most common treatments used by physiotherapists in the management of neck pain are hands-on techniques (manual therapy) and exercise. These traditional physiotherapy techniques need to be done in conjunction with advice and education, and the most important aspect of physiotherapy is teaching the person how to manage their own symptoms.

Neck pain is one of the most common associated symptoms of migraine, even more so than nausea. More than three quarters of people with migraine experience neck pain. Many experts in migraine believe that this neck pain is merely an extension of the migraine headache, and that the only way to successfully treat the neck pain is to treat the migraine.

Recent research has shown that palpation (touching or examining by hand) of the neck can reproduce a familiar head pain in people with migraine. This is interesting as it is thought that there may be a subgroup of people with migraine in whom the neck muscles and joints are acting as another trigger. The reason that neck pain is such a common symptom of migraine is due to the anatomical connections between nerves from the upper part of the neck, and those nerves from the head and face. Sensations such as pain from both areas are felt in the same area of the brain. This means that when someone has a migraine often the increased sensitivity of the nerves can extend to include increased sensitivity of the nerves of the upper neck, giving the sensation of pain in the neck area without there being any problem with the neck muscles or joints.

This anatomical link is also the reason why the neck can cause or worsen pain in the head. When somebody without a history of migraine has a pain in their neck which is connected to their head this is called cervicogenic headache. This has been the type of headache that most physiotherapists have concentrated their research on in the past, and this research has shown that physiotherapy treatment to the neck can help to relieve head pain. Usually this physiotherapy treatment involves:

o Hands-on treatment of the neck joints and muscles.
o Advice about posture correction.
o Exercises specifically formulated to improve movement or strength of neck and posture muscles.

Neck pain as a trigger of migraine is a newer concept. The physiotherapy management of neck pain when someone has migraine is more complex. There are people who get a lot of neck pain with their migraine but who will not improve with physiotherapy. Unfortunately sometimes these people waste a lot of time and money before they figure this out. However, there are also a number of people living with migraine whose neck muscles or joints are acting as a headache trigger and physiotherapy treatment should be part of their multi-disciplinary care.

How does a physiotherapist assess if the neck pain and migraine are related?

If you feel that your neck is a potential trigger to your migraine then the next step is to be assessed by a chartered physiotherapist who is specially trained in the treatment of headache and migraine. Most private physiotherapists have websites which would indicate if they have an interest in treating neck pain and headache. When you phone to make an appointment it would be wise to ask if they have ever treated someone with migraine before.

A physiotherapist will ask you questions about your neck pain and migraine and will use a hands-on assessment to determine if the neck is involved as a potential trigger for your migraine. The type of questions a physiotherapist may ask include questions about:

o Any previous neck injury.
o Relationship of headache to neck movements.
o Poor postures or awkward head positions.

A physiotherapist who treats headaches and migraine should have enough experience and expertise to confidently discuss your diagnosis of migraine, and to reassure you that there are no other potential more serious causes of headache. This is especially important if you have visited a private physiotherapist without being assessed by a doctor in the first instance.

The treatment of migraine is unique and the physiotherapist must take into account that your neck will only ever be one trigger. The 'avoidance' or management of this trigger requires a physiotherapy assessment and treatment specific to the neck problem. However, for overall successful migraine management all other triggers need to be recognised, such as:

o Hormonal changes.
o Changes in sleep pattern.
o Skipping meals.
o Certain foods.
o Dehydration.

An example of the kind of situation that a physiotherapist may commonly deal with is a person with a lifelong or family history of migraine, whose headaches get worse following a road traffic accident or due to longer hours sitting at a computer or desk.

The examination usually reveals head pain with neck movement or palpation of the upper neck joints and muscles. Other aspects of assessment include neck muscle strength and posture. The type of palpation commonly used by a physiotherapist on the spine is called 'Passive Accessory Intervertebral Movement', which means the joints in the neck are moved passively by the physiotherapist, usually while the person is lying down on a treatment bed. If you are not comfortable lying down, a version of this palpation can be done sitting.

There is a slight risk that a hands-on palpation like this can worsen your headache for a day or two following assessment. If this is the case, ensure you tell your physiotherapist on the following visit so that he or she will proceed more gently the next time. In particular a physiotherapist will be looking to see if the person feels a familiar pain in the head if they press on a particular neck muscle or joint. Lots of people can have tender muscles or stiff joints, but this alone does not implicate the neck as a source of head pain.

Frequently, an assessment alone will raise the physiotherapist's suspicion that the neck may be acting as a trigger, but unfortunately it is often only through a trial of treatment that you or the physiotherapist can be sure. A key message is that if you do not see some improvement in headache symptoms after three sessions of appropriate physiotherapy treatment, it is unlikely to help your symptoms.

Treatment of the neck in people with migraine and neck pain
The mainstay of treatment of neck pain related to migraine involves a combination of manual 'hands-on' therapy and exercises. At this point in time there is no quality research to support physiotherapy in the treatment of migraine; however, physiotherapists use the evidence available on other headache types such as cervicogenic headache to decide on which treatment to use.

Hands-on treatment techniques are focused specifically on stiff and tender areas of the neck, particularly those areas that have been found to reproduce a familiar head pain. If the source of pain is thought to be one of the neck muscles, the physiotherapist will likely look for tender areas in the muscle, commonly referred to as 'trigger points'. They will then use firm palpation of usually one finger over a 'trigger point' in an effort to desensitise the area. If a physiotherapist touches on one of these tender areas, it can be quite uncomfortable for the first few seconds; you should then feel that the intensity of discomfort reduces gradually over approximately one minute.

Some physiotherapists may offer to use a technique called dry needling to treat these tender 'trigger points'. Dry needling involves using an acupuncture needle instead of finger pressure over the trigger point. Do not worry if you don't like needles or if your physiotherapist does not offer this, as releasing the tightness with fingers or hands is likely to be beneficial too. In fact, the advantage of using hands instead of needles is that you can learn the technique yourself for use at home.

If the source of pain is deemed to be due to stiff neck joints the physiotherapist will likely use a technique called 'mobilisation' over the stiff area(s). This involves repeated movement of the joint in an effort to make it looser and less tender. Most physiotherapists will use their thumbs on one joint of the neck at a time, while you are lying face down on the treatment table.

The physiotherapist may carry out this mobilisation technique in one of two ways:

o The first is called 'oscillatory', where you will feel the pressure of their thumbs pulsing on and off in a rhythmical way.
o The second, called 'sustained', is where they press firmly with their thumb and do not release the pressure until after the discomfort has released (usually one minute).

It is also possible to have a similar treatment while you are lying face up. One way has not been shown to be superior to the other. There are slight advantages to using sustained holds while lying in face up position as you are more likely to be able to learn a similar technique yourself for use at home. There are even some mobilisation techniques that can be used in a sitting position. Make sure you tell your physiotherapist if you are more comfortable in one position compared to another.

Some physiotherapists are trained to use manipulation, similar to the techniques used by osteopaths and chiropractors. Manipulation is high-velocity thrusts beyond the physiological limit joint. There is no proven benefit for this technique over more gentle techniques, and manipulation has an additional risk to the important arteries in the neck that carry blood supply from the heart to the brain. The extreme end of this risk includes stroke and death, so it is recommended to ask your physiotherapist to use gentle, low-risk, hands-on techniques.

It is also highly recommended that you take an active approach to your own physiotherapy treatment. As there is no cure for migraine, you will need to learn to manage your neck pain in a similar way to managing any of your other potential triggers. In this way, any time you have a flare-up of neck pain you can self-treat instead of having to rush off to a physiotherapist.

Some of the treatment techniques a physiotherapist may show you include how to release out tender trigger points or 'knots' from certain muscles, or how to loosen up stiff neck joints with your own hands.

Home exercises often include exercises to stretch out any tightness and/or strengthen any weak muscles. Neck muscles can get weak or tight from sitting for long periods of time in a poor position, such as with the head jutting forward.

While there is no strong evidence of the 'perfect posture', your physiotherapist will likely also show you how to sit in an upright but comfortable position. Lots of people when they are told to 'sit up straight' adopt a strained or tense posture. It is a good skill to learn to be able to sit in an aligned position without any extra tension on any part of your body, including your neck. Some people who really struggle with this may be advised to consider a yoga or pilates class to help their posture awareness, to loosen up stiff areas of the body, and to get stronger in those muscles which can help to keep them upright but relaxed. These deep postural muscles are called our 'core' muscles. Looking at the body as a whole rather than just as a head on a neck can be beneficial if posture is thought to be a factor relating to the neck pain.

What do I do if physiotherapy treatment to the neck does not help my migraine symptoms?

Do not continue attending physiotherapy if there is not a significant improvement in your symptoms. Some improvement should be seen within three sessions, which will allow you to decide if you wish to continue using time, money, or energy to attend appointments. For significant improvements most people will generally need at least six sessions. Sometimes, people continue physiotherapy for much longer than this even though there is no improvement. Among other reasons, this can be due to a strong desire that the neck be identified as the main problem, as 'neck pain' can be an easier diagnosis to cope with than 'migraine'.

Just because the physiotherapist finds tenderness of your neck does not mean that your neck is a trigger for migraine, or that treatment aimed at the neck will help. People with migraine often get sensitised to lots of sensory information, such as:

o Noise.
o Smell.
o Bright lights or movements.

Being sensitive to pressure, pain, or touch on the neck may just be a symptom of your migraine, and not necessarily that the neck is the source of pain. In fact, for some people with severe migraine their neck may be so sensitive to touch that any attempt at physiotherapy makes them feel worse.

The best thing to do is to keep a detailed headache diary for at least one month before you start physiotherapy, and then continue to record your symptoms during your treatment. You may consider discontinuing physiotherapy if there is no positive significant change in:

o The number of days you are getting headache.
o The severity of your symptoms.
o The length of time that they last.

What if physiotherapy is not working for you?
Often physiotherapy alone is ineffective for a condition as complex as migraine. It may be that combined with the right lifestyle changes and medication the addition of physiotherapy can be beneficial, but alone it cannot help.

These other aspects of migraine management are covered in their appropriate chapters throughout this book and include:

o Having a regular sleep pattern.
o Eating regular meals.
o Staying hydrated.
o Practicing some relaxation or Mindfulness each day.
o Getting advice on preventative medication if you suffer from headache on more than fifteen days per month.
o Not using standard painkillers, anti-inflammatories or Triptans on more than ten days per month (to prevent medication overuse headache).

What do I do if physiotherapy treatment to the neck helps my symptoms?
If physiotherapy has successfully identified your neck as one of your migraine triggers, and a combination of hands-on treatment and exercise is helping, then ensure that you speak to your physiotherapist about teaching you how to self-manage your neck pain. You cannot keep attending physiotherapy for life, and if your migraine is a life-long condition you need self-management skills to manage this neck trigger as well as your other triggers.

Physiotherapy for dizziness in migraine
A migraine attack can also commonly include what are called vestibular symptoms, such as dizziness, head movement intolerance and unsteadiness, imbalance or disequilibrium. People with migraine often describe their disequilibrium as 'having just stepped off a boat'.

When the vestibular symptoms of migraine are very prominent, the condition may be classified as 'vestibular migraine'. Diagnostic criteria for vestibular migraine were added to the most recent version of the International Classification of Headache Disorders. These criteria outline that:

o A person must have a current or past history of migraine with or without aura.
o The vestibular symptoms must last between five and seventy-two hours.

At least 50% of the vestibular symptoms must be associated with migraineous features such as:

o Headache which is unilateral, pulsating and aggravated by routine physical activity.
o Photophobia (sensitivity to light) and phonophobia (sensitivity to sound, or visual aura).

Other symptoms that are commonly associated with vestibular migraine include:

o Nausea and vomiting.
o Susceptibility to motion sickness.
o Tinnitus.
o Fluctuating hearing loss, and aural (ear) fullness.

Vestibular rehabilitation has been proven to be effective for many different types of vestibular symptoms, such as those caused by unilateral vestibular loss. In the absence of high-quality studies relating to the management of dizziness in migraine, many physiotherapists offer vestibular rehabilitation to improve outcomes as part of multi-modal therapy or using more than one treatment approach. Similar to the management of neck pain in migraine, the physiotherapy management of dizziness symptoms in migraine is only likely to be beneficial when carried out in conjunction with lifestyle management and appropriate use of medications.

Only certain public and private physiotherapists are expert in this specific area of vestibular rehabilitation, so it is worth asking before you book yourself in. A physiotherapist will first carry out a full assessment to ascertain if any of your dizziness symptoms are related to an inner ear disorder, or if they appear to be part of your migraine symptoms.

Treatment will likely involve gaze-stability and balance exercises that you will carry out at home every day. One common type of gaze stability exercise is to focus on a single letter taped to a blank wall while you move your head left and right or up and down. Your physiotherapist will guide you as to the correct speed and correct amount of time to do this exercise or others that they prescribe. A common type of balance exercise is to practise standing in a narrow stance or even on one leg. Balance exercise must be carried out somewhere safe, as there is a risk of falling if you challenge your balance too much.

Some people find that these types of exercises can help their symptoms of dizziness or unsteadiness in the short term, but that the next time they get a migraine, their vestibular symptoms return. It is most likely that this type of rehabilitation will help you to feel less dizzy or unsteady in between migraine attacks, but it cannot stop your brain being sensitive during a migraine attack. Like all aspects of physiotherapy in migraine, one type of management done in isolation is rarely beneficial.

A suggested online resource for readers can be found at: www.severeheadacheexpert.com.

8

THE PSYCHOLOGY OF MIGRAINE

Dr Marie Murray

Marie Murray is a Clinical Psychologist, Psychotherapist and author. She is a Registered Psychologist, Registered Family Therapist, Member of the European Association for Psychotherapy and former Member of the Heads of Psychology Services in Ireland. Key posts in her clinical service over forty years have included Director of Psychology in St Vincent's Psychiatric Hospital, Dublin and Director of the Student Counselling Services in UCD. She was on the faculty of the Mater Family Therapy Training Programme, on the Academic Advisory Board of the CTYI at DCU and Course Director of the Masters in Psychotherapy at UL. A former member of the Irish Medical Council, she is currently on the Council of the Psychological Society of Ireland.

INTRODUCTION

Many people think that suffering from migraine is like having a bad headache. But as every chapter in this book confirms, migraine is a complex, disabling neurological disorder.

Migraine is also an extraordinarily extensive topic, so in this chapter I will focus on some of the primary psychological dimensions of the disorder for the child, adolescent and adult sufferer and I will outline a range of treatment options that have been found to be helpful.

HISTORICAL PERSPECTIVE

The psychological suffering of migraineurs has received insufficient attention until recent times. Although records of migraine reportedly date back almost 4,000 years, the condition itself was historically misunderstood, not least because disorders that physicians could not explain were categorised as 'hysterical'. The term 'hysteria' (from the Greek word for womb) was mainly reserved for 'women's' disorders and associated with uncontrollable emotional excess or trauma-based neurosis.

Sigmund Freud, father of psychoanalysis, famously suffered from 'migraine', yet by categorising his female patients' inexplicable physical complaints as those of 'hysterical', 'neurotic women' he contributed to the misunderstanding of migraine. Of course, the technology of his time did not provide the psychoneurological insights we have now but the residue of such thinking still lingers in public consciousness. Clichéd jokes about women 'having a headache' to avoid sex is one example (although coital headache primarily affects men). This may also reflect the 3:1 incidence of migraine in women, or that now outdated notion of 'hysteria' but regardless of their origin, myths about migraine can make migraine not only psychologically difficult for women, but add to men's silence about their migraine too.

PSYCHOLOGY OF MIGRAINE

For the estimated half a million migraine sufferers in Ireland, thirty thousand of whom may have chronic migraine, life is exceptionally difficult. Chronic migraine is a pattern of having migraine on fifteen or more days every month, so it is not surprising that many migraineurs become psychologically overwhelmed, anxious and depressed by their migraine as it intrudes on their happiness, their relationships, their family life, their social lives, their careers and their overall capacity to cope.

Migraine also has significant psychological aspects because those who suffer from migraine spend considerable amounts of time in pain. Not only is the pain disabling when it occurs, but in between migraine attacks migraineurs spend time trying to manage their lives so as to reduce the frequency, severity, intensity and the duration of attacks and the impact of their migraine on their own life and on the lives of other people.

Additionally, the period between migraine episodes, known as the 'interictal' period, is not necessarily migraine free because many migraineurs may experience below the radar kinds of pain and heightened sensitivity (allodynia) such as sensitivity to light, sound, touch, weather and surroundings. With little or no reprieve for chronic migraineurs, psychological distress is to be expected. Understanding and attending to the interrelated physical, psychological and social distress of migraine is crucial to coping.

BIOPSYCHOSOCIAL APPROACH TO MIGRAINE

What is called the biopsychosocial approach to migraine recognises the connection between the biological, the psychological and the social factors in chronic illness. No aspect can be treated in isolation and migraine is a fine example of how these three factors overlap and interact, each influencing the other in migraine sufferers.

It can sometimes be difficult to determine which came first – the condition or depression – because with disorders such as migraine, when there is co-morbidity with depression, anxiety and other enduring mental health challenges, people who suffer from migraine are understandably wary of their migraine being viewed as 'psychological'. This may be why many migraineurs hide their migraine and talk about it as little as possible. Many also fear having their episodes of migraine misinterpreted as attention seeking, as exaggerated or as an excuse to extricate themselves from activities in which they do not want to engage.

We need to recognise the psychological stress that physical illnesses cause because chronic conditions by their nature take a toll on the individual and the entire network of people that surround a sufferer. Suffering causes stress, which in turn exacerbates suffering, in a circular, ever-revolving and distressing pattern for migraineurs as they await the next migraine episode.

COMPLEXITY OF MIGRAINE

Complex factors make up the experience of being a migraineur. These include the search for diagnosis; migraine's unpredictability, its chronicity; the severity of pain; the ongoing stress; the danger of being given an identity as 'disabled' and the compromises in family, workplace and social life. Migraine is a psychological challenge because of the following:

Diagnosis
o   The 'invisibility' of the condition and the frequent delay in diagnosis.
o   The extent to which diagnosis is dependent on the personal account by sufferers of their subjective experience and migraine patterns.
o   The adjustment reactions to diagnosis. There may be grief about time lost before diagnosis or there may be disappointment that management of the condition rather than cure is offered. In a world where advances in medicine lead us to expect cure rather than living with illness this can be an initial psychological blow and it can also take time to adjust to the realisation that treatment requires a personal, active and collaborative relationship between psychologist and migraineur.

Pain
o   The pain factor is high in migraine. Research shows that those who live with chronic pain conditions or the ongoing threat of pain, in addition to being more prone to anxiety and depression, also suffer the stress of the condition on cognition, thinking and memory in addition to sleep disturbance, feelings of frustration, hopelessness and other mental health stresses.

o When attacks of migraine occur there is uncertainty about how they will progress in terms of pain, intensity and duration. Migraineurs wonder if they will be in misery for an hour, a few hours, a day or a few days.

o Each bout begs the question: how long will it last and how bad will it be?

o The excruciating pain of cluster headaches are so severe that they are described as 'like a hot poker to the eye'. More common in men these are the headaches that reduce grown men to tears of desperation, yet there is little public recognition of this.

Stress

o The stress of trying to live a normal life with an intrusive condition.

o The aftermath or 'interictal' stress, after an attack and before the next episode because even a low-lying threatening level between attacks is psychologically challenging.

o Hypervigilance for the next episode – migraineurs are always on the lookout for the tiniest signs that another migraine is on the way, which can contribute to the onset of episodes.

o Migraine is the penultimate saboteur of plans and because it strikes unexpectedly it is virtually impossible to plan ahead. The entire family may be on alert before important family events, which causes everyone stress.

o The association between migraine and stroke causes worry and the experience of aura can be particularly frightening as people may think they are having a stroke.

Identity

o There are identity difficulties in having a chronic condition, and feeling defined in terms of it.

o Societal and cultural misunderstanding about migraine can cut into psychological well-being and self-esteem.

o This is allied to a sense of stigma that sufferers still report. Many men avoid admitting that they suffer from migraine and many women feel that they are psychologically categorised once they say that they are migraineurs.

o Migraineurs are often reluctant to make complaints in relationships and in the workplace for fear of being regarded as 'complainers'.

o Some migraineurs feel inexplicable guilt when an attack commences, as if they have either done something to cause it, or omitted to do something to avoid it.

In summary, migraine is a condition whose presence is never absent from consciousness, whose arrival is often dramatic and incapacitating, whose invasion of personal life is extreme, whose intrusion into the family is upsetting and whose constraints in the workplace can strain relationships with colleagues and jeopardise careers. However, it is important to point out that from the psychological perspective, even when there are not cures, there are always 'solutions' to be found in the form of therapeutic interventions, which will be discussed later.

MIGRAINE AND CHILDREN

If adults, who can at least articulate and understand what is happening to them, feel upset and misconstrued by migraine, then when migraine appears in 'disguise' in childhood it can be exceptionally stressful for parents and children. The main problems for children arise from the following:

o Being misunderstood. A child often does not know what is happening, is unlikely to be able to put words on symptoms and may only be able to act out pain behaviourally.

o The danger of a psychological label. Children's migraine symptoms can be misinterpreted as the child being of a difficult angry or irritable temperament rather than being understood as a physical complaint.

o Migraine's abdominal presentation is open to misconstrual because tummy upset is usually defined as a psychological distress signal in children.

o Having to stay indoors to avoid light and noise adds to a child's sense of difference.

o The child may have the embarrassment of nausea and vomiting symptoms – for example at a party or in school.

o At school, being unable to play with friends at break time can make cementing friendships more difficult.

o Periods of poor concentration, inattention and incapacity caused by migraine can make a child appear to be less able intellectually or academically. Any falling behind reduces academic self-esteem.

o There may be avoidance of strenuous play, attendance at PE or problems on school tours.

o Children feel everything with visceral sensitivity and intensity and so the physical experience of pain can be more traumatic for children than for people at later developmental stages.

o The additional sensitivity (allodynia) of migraine can mean that it hurts the child to have their head touched or hair brushed. Even clothing labels, 'scratchy' fabrics and bed linens can be annoying. If adults are not aware of this the child can seem to be cranky.

o Unconsciously avoiding triggers such as at funfairs: roller coasters, bumpers, the big wheel; this creates the embarrassment of vertigo or being seen as cowardly by peers.

o Feeling different to friends when the one and most important aspiration for every child is to be the same as everyone else.

Everything that impinges on childhood or on how a child is perceived has psychological implications. The identification of migraine in children and its timely treatment are important to psychosocial development too.

MIGRAINE AND ADOLESCENTS

Adolescence is about youth, vibrancy, energy and purpose. It is not about having an intrusive, potentially chronic condition. Adolescents who suffer from migraine do so at an especially sensitive and challenging developmental stage. Any disadvantage at this time is heightened psychologically because it is a time when peer opinions matter. It is also a time associated with significant mood variations which add to the psychological complexity of migraine at this developmental stage. Traditionally the core task of adolescence is the search for identity so that having a migraine identity foisted upon the young person is distressing. Developmentally the following are also of note:

o Lifestyle triggers are probably at their peak in adolescence and young adulthood in terms of late hours, screen time, disrupted sleep, socialising in groups and in high-decibel noisy venues! All wonderful when young – but a nightmare for young migraineurs.

o Education can suffer through absence from school and problems with concentration and retention when attending. In fact, headaches rank third among illness-related causes of school absenteeism.

o Exam stress can trigger attack.

o Making applications for special accommodation for exams can be a dilemma for the young person as to whether they want to be identified or not as requiring special treatment.

o Any reference to, or definition of them in terms of 'disability' can distress young people.

o Oppositional defiance difficulties can get displaced and acted out in non-compliance with managing migraine.

o Alcohol can be an issue if there is pressure to drink from peers, especially because alcohol can be a trigger for migraine.

o Impulsivity, the wish to comply with friends allied to poor capacity to make judgements of risk, can make migraine management difficult.

o   The developmental strive for independence during adolescence can hinder compliance and self-management.
o   In any situation of family conflict there is the risk that this can be displaced onto migraine, making it harder to manage.
o   There may be an 'instinctive' avoidance of sport, especially contact sports that might trigger migraine. This can exclude migraineurs from the excitement of competitive sport.
o   For migraineurs, missing the continuity of interaction with the peer group, even temporarily, brings challenges. This is an under-discussed dimension to migraine – the generalised and social anxiety it may trigger.
o   Having to miss social events can also trigger social anxiety, which can escalate into social phobia in already sensitive young people.
o   Adolescent boys can feel embarrassed to have a 'headache' and loneliness has been associated with headache in adolescents.
o   Anything that differentiates a young person from peers brings the risk of being bullied. Sadly migraine is no exception. This may leave the young person hiding their migraine, hiding being bullied or acting out their distress in ways that bring further negativity towards them.
o   The incompatibility of some career choices with migraine is upsetting.
o   All adolescent eyes are on the future and with a chronic disorder the future can look less positive.

MIGRAINE AND MARITAL AND FAMILY RELATIONSHIPS

When the brain coordinates go awry, headache may or may not be on the way, but an 'episode' has begun and life is on hold until it ends. This is one of the great causes of distress for migraineurs, their partners and children.

In fact, many partners of migraineurs say that they suffer from chronic vicarious migraine, because they live 'with' the condition on a daily basis and their own lives are circumscribed by it. The impact on the family and the guilt that many migraineurs feel at having to restrict the life of their partner or children or let them down is a major stressor. This can also trigger anxiety, depression, medication misuse or overuse by migraineurs who are desperate to stave off an attack when important family events are imminent. Here are some common negative effects of migraine on the family:

o There is strain around family events if a family member is frequently absent.
o For migraineur and partner there is additional strain on the relationship when couples are expected to attend events together.
o It is difficult for migraineurs to volunteer for school-related activities such as sports days, car pools and play dates.
o Children may not understand why a parent has to avoid events
that 'all the other parents' attend.
o Entering a darkened room, being excluded from contact with a parent
and being prohibited from making noise can be hard for children.
o Children hate to see a parent prostrate with pain and can worry
that a parent might die.
o If adolescents are going through a difficult or oppositional stage,
migraine can worsen family dynamics.
o Family holidays may be compromised because stress, fatigue,
change in routine and travel can be triggers.
o The genetic component in some migraines adds to family concern.

MIGRAINE AND THE WORKPLACE

Think of all the possible occupations a person may have; then imagine performing those occupations while suffering a migraine attack! Imagine gearing up for a busy sales period; making appointments that you may not be able to keep; scheduling presentations that you will never give; planning seminars you might not attend; lecturing through a fog of pain; having to attend staff meetings without being able to concentrate.

Imagine driving a bus, train, taxi or patrol car, or rushing to a fire. Imagine sitting at a computer with its screen flashing all day. Think about working in a crèche or teaching a class of thirty children with a crashing headache. Imagine feeling nauseous, confused or disoriented; flinching at every sound, squinting to block out painful light, about to throw up and with a body that has become alien and unco-ordinated. Think of a brain of jumbled wires where even thinking and speaking is problematic. That is migraine – which is why workplace issues for migraineurs include the following:

o Attempts to work through an episode may not only extend the severity and duration of migraine, but in certain professions could lead to dangerous errors given how cognition, attention, competence and capacity are compromised during an attack.

o Strain on relationships with colleagues is always a possibility if the migraineur appears to have unequal time away from work.

o Not only is workplace absenteeism an issue, but presenteeism (being there but dysfunctional) can also cause problems.

o Confidence about seeking career advancement is diminished.

o The limitation placed on choice of careers is a source of grief for those with aspirations to 'migraine-unfriendly' careers.

o The definition of 'disability' in relation to migraine is still being clarified from the employment law perspective, so migraineurs may not be confident about their entitlements in the workplace.

o Some migraineurs only look for part-time work so that they can juggle hours to 'repay' time taken off with migraine.

MIGRAINE AND INTERVENTIONS

We have seen the impact of migraine on people's lives in a range of contexts, all of which highlight the need for cultural, educational, family and organisational support and the importance of multidisciplinary interventions so that migraineurs' psychological needs are attended to.

There is a case to be made for all migraineurs having access to psychological support. This would ultimately be cost-effective because there is significant evidence that psychology is an essential component of the biopsychosocial approach to migraine because of the following:

o The manner in which the biological, psychological and social dimensions of migraine interact.
o Psychological support when the individual type, trajectory, triggers and pattern of migraine are initially being tracked.
o Specific intervention with regard to fear-generated Medication Overuse Headaches (MOH).
o Evidence of the impact of migraine on mental health and well-being especially when there is co-morbidity of psychological factors that could impact on compliance with treatment.
o The bidirectionality between migraine, mood, anxiety, sleep disorders and depression and other enduring mental health challenges.
o The research that suggests that major depression is significantly more common in migraine sufferers than in the general population shows how crucial psychological intervention is in helping people cope.
o The extreme distress of 'cluster' headaches requires sustained support.

Psychologists have an important role in assessing and encouraging collaboration between migraineurs and professionals and in teaching techniques for the control of stress and pain symptoms. These include self-management techniques as well as more formal psychotherapy interventions.

SELF-MANAGEMENT TECHNIQUES

Lifestyle Adjustment
o Keeping a personal migraine diary reveals the unique pattern of a person's migraine and shows what helps or hinders management of it.

o Monitoring personal progress on MIDAS (Migraine Disability Assessment) the HIT (Headache Impact Test) and other relevant questionnaires that facilitate measuring migraine's impact.

o Managing diet, sleep, activity, work, social schedules, stressors and relaxation time all contribute towards self-management.

o Acknowledging 'let down' migraine, which happens after a period of specific stress; tracking it and learning to pace activities to avoid it.

o Recognising when support is needed; seeking and accepting it.

o Building enjoyable activities into routine as a psychological counterbalance to the frustration of having a chronic condition. In other words, if you are burdened by times of pain make sure you schedule as many good times as possible in between.

Positive Affirmations

o Research shows the value of people having formal training in positive affirmations. These are selective repetitive positive statements that a person consciously makes to him or herself – for example 'the pain is going', 'I can cope'. This simple self-hypnosis technique is easy to learn, efficient and effective.

Minimal-Therapist-Contact-Treatment (MTCT)

o The value of self-management through MTCT cannot be overemphasised. This means that migraineurs learn about their own specific migraine and identify, in detail, everything that aggravates or alleviates it for progressive personal migraine management.

FORMAL INTERVENTIONS

Psychological Interventions

o Cognition, emotions and pain experiences change the way the brain processes information but there is evidence through fMRI (technology showing the brain in action) that psychological interventions assist in pain management.

o Shared circuitry between areas of the brain that process pain and those that process emotions, attention and stress suggests that altering the signals in one area may help the other, which is why psychological interventions, regularly undertaken, can reduce pain and increase coping skills.

o Given the bidirectionality of distress and migraine, psychotherapeutic discussion with a professional about past and present life events and stressors may help self-management.

o Experiences of pain generate anticipation of pain, which increase frequency and may intensify the next pain experience. Psychotherapy has a role in stopping that negative cycle of hypervigilance for the next attack.

o Psychotherapy also helps sufferers to shift the locus of control from exclusive dependence on medicine and medication to recognising the importance of their own internal control of their condition.

o Psychotherapy also supports those who do not respond to conventional therapies.

Systemic Psychotherapy and Family Therapy

o Systemic Psychotherapy is that in which therapists work collaboratively with migraineurs to analyse every aspect of their lives, relationships, family, work and social contexts to help them consider all lifestyle options, treatment priorities, psychological management and communication with others about their condition. Marital and family dynamics that have been altered by migraine are specifically addressed by this model.

Autogenic Training

o Autogenic relaxation training literally teaches the body to respond to what you tell it to do and is quick and easy to learn. Regular autogenic relaxation systematically reduces muscle tension caused by pain and stress, for example, by imagining each part of the body in turn becoming heavy, warm and relaxed it can also help induce sleep.

Biofeedback
o   Biofeedback is an approach that uses technology to systematically train the body to control stress and the person can hear, see and feel themselves succeed in doing so. Thermal Biofeedback, based on body temperature, has been found to be particularly helpful for migraine sufferers.
o   Biofeedback 'games' are appropriate for children and there are adolescent versions that make the therapy entertaining.
o   What is called Psychophysiological Insomnia – basically a hyperactive, hyperaroused, 'worrying' brain that finds it hard to shut down, even for sleep – can be helped through biofeedback to learn shut-down strategies.

Progressive Muscle Relaxation
o   Training in how to progressively relax the body, for example tensing muscles and releasing them and noting the difference is effective in 'unclenching' the body.
o   It can be useful to rate tension levels from 0-100 with 0 represeing no tension and 100 representing unbearable tension and then monitor at what point along the scale you are when engaged in different activities throughout the day.

Acceptance and Commitment Therapy (ACT)
o   ACT is based on training in acceptance of what is out of a person's control while committing to action that will improve quality of life for migraineurs.

Cognitive Behaviour Therapy (CBT)
o   Cognitive behaviour therapy is an evidence-based approach which involves training in how to think and act. It has been found to be effective in headache management by reducing stress, distress and catastrophising, severity of headaches and medication use. It increases resilience through cognitive strategies worked out between psychologist and migraineur, which are plans on how

to think about, behave towards and cope with migraine. Actively building strategies into each day is therapeutic, as in this Rescue Plan which takes the acronym RESCUE as a useful reminder to:

R – Remain Calm
E – Escape from known triggers
S – Stay away from stress
C – Carry migraine medication at all times
U – Use relaxation exercises
E – Eat and sleep on schedule

SUMMARY

Despite all the complex dimensions of migraine, how dreadfully people suffer and how intensely migraine can intrude on life, it cannot be repeated too often that there is always hope. There are many ways of managing migraine, only some of which I have touched upon above. When people understand their own migraine, make appropriate and timely use of medication, engage in flexible self-management, collaborate with professional support, undertake lifestyle adjustment, do systemic and family analysis of their situation and choose from the range of techniques and psychological strategies to deal with their migraine it can become manageable, with good reason to hope.

Continued research, expanded service provision, accessing the expertise of the MAI and calling for the provision of specific, dedicated psychological services for migraineurs will increase hope for those who have suffered courageously for such a long time.

REFERENCES

o Bird, J. and Pinch, C. (2002), *Autogenic therapy: self-help for mind and body*, Dublin: Newleaf.

o Hayes, S.C., Strosahl, K.C., and Wilson, K.G. (2012), *Acceptance and Commitment Therapy: The Process and Practice of Mindful Change*, New York: Guilford Press.

o Jette, N., Patten, S., Williams, J., Becker, W., and Wiebe, S, 'Comorbidity of migraine and psychiatric disorders: A national population-based study', *Headache*, 2008;48:501–516.

o Lipchik, G.L, Holroyd, K.A., and Nash, J.M. (2002), *Cognitive-Behavioral Management of Recurrent Headache Disorders: A Minimal-Therapist-Contact Approach*, in Turk, D.C. and Gatchel, R.J. (eds), *Psychological approaches to pain management* (2nd edn), New York: Guilford (This also contains the RESCUE Plan above).

o McGoldrick, M., Carter, B., and Garcia-Preto, N. (2013), *The Expanded Family Life Cycle: Individual, Family, and Social Perspectives* (4th edn).

o Olesen, J. (Chairman), 'Headache Classification Subcommittee of the International Headache Society. The International Classification of Headache Disorders: 2nd edition', *Cephalalgia*, 2004;24(suppl 1):9–160.

o Sexton, T.L., and Lebow, J. (2016), *Handbook of Family Therapy*, New York: Routledge.

o Woods, B.L., 'A developmental biopsychosocial approach to the treatment of chronic illness in children and adolescents', in Mikesell, R.H. et al. (1995) (eds), *Integrating Family Therapy: Handbook of Psychology and Systems Theory* (435–455), Washington DC: American Psychological Association.

9

MIGRAINE IN CHILDREN

Dr Deirdre Peake

Deirdre Peake is a Paediatric Neurologist with a specialist interest in epilepsy and tic disorders. She sees a wide variety of childhood neurological illnesses including headache up to the age of sixteen years. She qualified from University College Dublin in 1994 with an honours degree and undertook General Paediatric training in Dublin. She became a national grid trainee in the UK, where she obtained her Certificate of Completion of Specialist Training in Paediatric Neurology (CCST) in 2006. She initially worked as a Paediatric Neurologist in Birmingham Children's Hospital, and since 2007 holds a permanent post as a Consultant in Paediatric Neurology in Royal Belfast Hospital for Sick Children, Belfast.

INTRODUCTION

Headache in children is a very common but under-recognised and underdiagnosed disorder. Studies show up to 2 out of 3 of children are reported to have one or more headaches in a twelve-month period and approximately 25% of adolescents suffer weekly headaches. They can occur on their own (primary headache) or as a result of another condition (secondary headache).

Headache is sometimes a cause for concern, and should be brought to the attention of a medical practitioner in order to eliminate other more serious conditions. The 'Headsmart' campaign (www.headsmart.org.uk) highlights different symptoms at specific ages that would prompt a more urgent medical referral. It is important to remember however that the majority of recurrent headaches in childhood are either tension-type headaches or migraines and are not associated with an underlying structural lesion in the brain.

DIAGNOSING MIGRAINE IN CHILDREN

An estimated 10% of children suffer from migraine – that's over 100,000 children in Ireland alone. The most common type of migraine in children is called 'migraine without aura'. The warning signs that sometimes come before the migraine, such as disturbed vision, strange taste or smells, or wobbliness, are referred to as an 'aura'. Diagnosing migraine without an aura in children can be difficult as it may manifest differently than in adults.

There are no hard and fast rules, but the following differences would not be atypical:

o Attacks are usually shorter in children (usually less than twenty-four hours but greater than one hour).
o Headache is not as severe.
o Headache may be on both sides of head rather than on one side.
o Gastrointestinal symptoms (for example, stomach ache) are usually more prominent in children.
o Equally prominent in boys before puberty. Thereafter, it is three times more common in girls.

If you feel your child may have migraine there are a few useful steps to take:

o Encourage your child to draw a picture of the headache if they are unable to verbalise it.
o Keep a diary of how frequently they occur, the length of time the headaches last, a description of the type of headache (examples such as thumping, pounding, tight band, sharp, knife-like can be given).

o Where in the head is the headache? Point with a finger to demonstrate.
o Note the time of the day the headache occurs and if anything makes the headache better or worse.
o Document if there are any associated factors such as vomiting, visual disturbances, photophobia or phonophobia (unable to tolerate light or noise).

The above information will enable the medical practitioner to identify if the characteristics are in keeping with paediatric migraine. A diagnosis of migraine may be made with the assistance of the International Headache Society (modified for children as they can be too specific and not sensitive enough) and by following 'Headaches in over 12s: diagnosis and management NICE guidelines [CG150]'.

Like in adults, the causes of migraine in children are thought to include many factors and are complex in nature. Environmental factors that can trigger a migraine attack include a change in climate or weather (such as a change in humidity or temperature), a change in altitude or barometric pressure, high winds, travelling, or a change in routine. Other environmental triggers include a bright or flickering light (sunlight reflections, glare, fluorescent lighting, television, or movies), extremes of heat and sound, and intense smells or vapours. They can also be aggravated or provoked by emotional/psychological stressors.

MIGRAINE EQUIVALENTS IN CHILDREN

Children can also present with a group of symptoms that does not include a headache at all. Instead, symptoms such as stomach ache, loss of appetite, nausea and vomiting may be the major part of a child's attack, making migraine harder to recognise in children. This is known as abdominal migraine and usually it evolves into more typical migraine after puberty. The abdominal pain can be dull, sore or intense and is usually located around the middle of the abdomen around the navel. Other symptoms such as vertigo (benign paroxysmal vertigo) and head-tilt (benign paroxysmal torticollis) can be variants of childhood migraine.

DOES MY CHILD NEED AN MRI SCAN?

The majority of children do not need to have any neuroimaging performed. In general, imaging is performed if there is anything abnormal found on clinical examination or if another cause of the headache is suspected.

WHY TAKE HEADACHE IN CHILDREN SERIOUSLY?

o The child's school performance may decline or it may result in significant school absence.
o Headaches can be debilitating, affecting the child's ability to participate in activities and social events.
o Relationships with friends and other family members can be affected.
o Migraine may be indicative of other trouble in the child's life such as lack of sleep, poor diet, stress, depression, or other illness.

Recent studies show that children with chronic headache are reported to have a worse quality of life compared to other chronic illnesses such as asthma or diabetes (Kernick D., Campbell J., *Cephalagia*, 2008).

MIGRAINE TRIGGERS IN CHILDREN

Trigger factors are frequently reported by children and adolescents with migraine: 'Triggers are factors that, alone or in combination, induce headache in susceptible individuals.' They are important in migraine management since their avoidance may result in a better control of the disorder. A recent study in 2012 by L. Vallee et al. ('Headache Pain,' Jan 2012; 13(1): 61–65) showed that the most common individual trigger was stress (75.5% of patients), followed by lack of sleep (69.6%), warm climate (68.6%) and video games (64.7%). Other triggers can include:

o Certain foods, for example cheese, citrus fruits, chocolate, fizzy drinks or preserved meats.
o Missed meals. In some cases a light snack before any extra activity could be all that is needed to prevent a migraine developing, as it is important to maintain a constant blood sugar level.
o Excessive physical exercise.
o Flickering lights such as fluorescent tube lighting, TV flicker or flashing images.

HOW TO MANAGE CHILDHOOD MIGRAINE

For children/young people
Maintaining a diary for up to three months to help establish patterns and to identify certain triggers may be helpful. Preventative measures and lifestyle changes may eliminate or decrease the number of attacks to avoid the need for prescribed drug therapies. Helpful changes may include:

o Regular meals.
o Regular sleep.
o Regular exercise and rest.
o Avoidance of caffeine.
o Adequate hydration – drinking plenty of water.
o Trigger avoidance identified in your diary.
o Talking to someone about your stressors.
o If you have been prescribed medicine, try to make sure it is always to hand.
o Keep a migraine ID card that you can hand to someone if you're unable to communicate.

For additional information and help go to the Migraine Association of Ireland's children's website.

For Parents

If the symptoms are noticed early a child can often sleep off the pain of migraine. Non-pharmacological management techniques include relaxation exercises, stress management, biofeedback and behavioural therapies. These therapies can greatly reduce the frequency of attacks. Although there is no conclusive evidence that reflexology is effective, many find it helpful, and ten treatments over 5–8 weeks may be worth trying if no other remedies work.

If your child is about to have an attack, a mild painkilling drug such as ibuprofen should be given as soon as possible (in soluble form as this is more quickly absorbed). Aspirin should be avoided due to its association with a rare condition called Reye's Syndrome (see Glossary). Nausea or vomiting can be countered with an anti-nausea drug, which can be bought over the counter; it should be taken about fifteen minutes before the painkiller.

Further advice

o Use your GP – get the correct diagnosis and have other possible causes of headache ruled out.

o Be prepared for an attack – if applicable, the child's medication should be to hand and given early in the attack.

o Learn to recognise migraine patterns and help your child to spot the early signs of an attack and learn to know when an attack might be about to happen.

o Tell the school principal and teacher; if there is a school nurse, inform them as well, especially if the child's attention or attendance might be affected.

o Reassure your child and support them.

o Help your child to establish regular sleeping and eating habits.

o Go to the MAI website for further information, support and advice (www.migraine.ie).

For teachers and others at school

The school principal, class teacher and/or school nurse should be informed of a child's susceptibility to migraine. This will ensure that proper action is taken in the event of an attack. It will also minimise disruption to a child's school routine.

Most schools co-operate very well with whatever treatment has been suggested to parents. Teachers/nurses may prefer to 'hold' younger children's medication and give it on request. It may be appropriate for older children to carry their own medication and take an emergency supply of appropriate tablets when necessary.

Every effort should be made to retain a normal routine and, where possible, avoid having to send the child home from school. Teachers can help students by being aware of symptoms and treatments. While learning themselves, teachers can also teach the rest of the class about how to recognise, react to and help during a migraine attack.

o Learn to recognise the signs.
o Contact the nurse if the school has one.
o Remove the student to a quiet, dark room if possible. This alone can sometimes abort an attack.
o If the student carries medication, give it as early as possible in the attack.
o If necessary, contact the student's parents or guardians.
o Self-help measures such as a short sleep or applying a cool pack can also help.
o If nothing above works, consider sending the pupil home.
o If in an emergency situation, or the parents/guardians cannot be contacted, call the child's GP.

TREATMENTS FOR A CHILD WITH MIGRAINE

There are two types of medicine:
o Reliever – these treatments are used during or at the beginning of a headache.

o Preventive – these medicines are taken every day to prevent headaches from occurring.

Infrequent attacks in children usually require conservative self-help approaches only. Discuss possible treatment options with your GP.

Reliever
Acute treatments are used to treat an attack once the symptoms of the attack have begun.

o Ibuprofen is readily available and inexpensive, making it an excellent first choice for migraine treatment.
o Triptans, the migraine-specific prescription drugs, are suitable options for children and adolescents when ibuprofen has failed to provide pain freedom or headache relief. They are generally prescribed by a paediatrician/paediatric neurologist. Minor unwanted side effects like taste disturbance, nasal symptoms, dizziness, fatigue, low energy, nausea, or vomiting are reported ('Drugs for the acute treatment of migraine in children and adolescents', Cochrane review, 2016).
o Anti-emetics are useful to relieve nausea and vomiting. They should be administered with caution and under medical supervision.

Preventive
Preventative medical therapy is rarely recommended for children. Regular preventative therapy may be justified (usually on a short two- or three-month trial period) if migraine attacks are very frequent, distressing or causing a significant impact on the child's quality of life. Following advice from a GP on the positive and negative aspects of treatment options, parents can decide on the best management solutions for their child. Some of the standard medications used to prevent migraine in adults are also used in children, for example Pizotifen, Beta blockers (propranolol), topirimate, sodium valproate, amitriptyline and flunarazine are used in children. Flunarizine is a

type of drug known as a calcium channel blocker thought to be most helpful in the adolescent age group and most effective in preventing migraine. It is an unlicensed drug.

Keep a note of any changes you or your child notice that you think might be a side effect of the medication. The most commonly reported side effects are drowsiness and weight gain. Record them in a migraine diary and report back to the doctor if necessary.

Complementary treatment
Some people find complementary treatments such as yoga therapy and biofeedback helpful. For further information visit www.migraine.ie. Learning how to cope with headache pain, using relaxation, stress management and guided imagery, can also be helpful.

Some good news
For most people, migraines improve or end by their late teens.

10

PROTECTING CHRONIC MIGRAINE SUFFERERS IN THEIR EMPLOYMENT: THE ROLE FOR LAW

Dr Caoimhín MacMaoláin

Dr Caoimhín MacMaoláin is an Associate Professor of Law and Fellow of Trinity College Dublin. His research primarily focuses on national, European Union and international Food Law, and he has published two books on this subject with Hart: Bloomsbury. He has previously undertaken research on the employment rights of migraineurs with the European Headache Alliance.

INTRODUCTION

As we know, migraine affects a very significant portion of the population, and consequently a large percentage of the workforce also. According to the World Health Organisation (WHO) Global Burden of Disease Study, updated in 2013, migraine is the sixth highest cause of years lived with disability. Headache disorders collectively were third highest. European and American studies have shown that between 6–8% of men and 15–18% of women experience migraine each year. Headache disorders tend to be most troublesome in the years from late teens to early fifties, therefore decreasing productivity during those years.

Migraine, as a result, also imposes a financial cost to society from lost working hours and reduced levels of productivity. In the United Kingdom, for example, it is estimated that 25 million working or school/education days are lost each year to migraine, extending to 190 million lost workdays across the EU. The European Headache Alliance has previously estimated that migraine costs the European economy €27 billion annually in reduced productivity. The WHO puts this figure at up to £140 billion globally.

According to the Migraine Association of Ireland, migraineurs miss up to an average of 4.5 days of work annually at a cost of €252 million to the Irish economy. Employment laws must be interpreted and applied in a manner that protects those who are temporarily unable to carry out work while suffering from the symptoms of migraine. They must also be devised and applied in a way that reduces the impact of this disorder on the economy, by creating working environments that minimise the potential triggers for an attack, where appropriate. Employment laws, and the rights available to employees that stem from these, are set out in a range of international, European Union and Irish documents and legislation.

There are two key aspects to any examination of what additional employment rights may be available to migraineurs in their workplace:

The first is establishing whether migraine can be considered as a 'disability', even a temporary one, which would bring the migraineur within the scope of the relevant EU and Irish employment equality laws.

The second is then to establish what additional rights may exist for the covered migraineur, and what limitations may legitimately be placed on the implementation of these allowances or accommodations by employers.

EMPLOYMENT LAW IN IRELAND

The majority of new employment laws protecting workers in Ireland now come directly from developments at European Union level. Guarantees are set out in the EU Treaty that measures will be devised and implemented that protect workers in their employment, including setting standards designed to eliminate exclusion, on whatever grounds, from the workforce. The main EU legislative initiative designed to meet these Treaty commitments is the Equal Treatment

Directive ('the Directive'). This is transposed into Irish law in the Employment Equality Acts.

Traditionally, the principle of equal treatment in European Union law has been primarily concerned with eliminating discrimination between men and women. However, as EU law has developed, so too has legislative recognition that other forms of discrimination exist in the workplace. These are accounted for in the Directive, which extends anti-discrimination rules to include discrimination based on disability. While suffering from migraine should not be considered a 'disability' as such, there are occasions when attacks may lead to symptoms that temporarily 'disable' the migraineur. When this happens, aspects of the relevant employment legislation should be applied to accommodate and protect the sufferer of chronic migraine symptoms.

DEFINING 'DISABILITY'

Before it can be established that the protections set out in the Equal Treatment Directive and the Employment Equality Acts apply to migraineurs, it must first be established whether or not chronic migraine can be considered a 'disability' under the law. Unhelpfully, the Equal Treatment Directive does not contain any definition of 'disability'. This could leave those suffering from conditions such as migraine in an uncertain legal position. Until the European Court of Justice or the legislative institutions set a definition, it is really up to each individual Member State to determine who will be covered by the disability provisions of the Equal Treatment Directive.

When determining just who may be covered by the protection set out in the EU Directive, the European Court of Justice has provided that three conditions must be met for a person to be considered 'disabled' in employment law:

o There is a limitation resulting from physical, mental or psychological impairments.

o The limitation hinders the participation of the person in professional life.

o It is probable that the limitation will last for a long time.

No criteria are set, however, for any of these general conditions, leaving it unclear as to whether an individual's condition can be considered a 'disability'. This leads to a lack of legal certainty in ascertaining what protection or accommodation may be legally available for those suffering from neurological conditions such as chronic migraine. We must therefore look to domestic law to ascertain who may be covered by these provisions of the Directive.

In Irish legislation 'disability' is defined as including 'the malfunction [...] of a part of a person's body' and/or 'a condition, illness or disease which affects a person's thought processes, [...] emotions or judgement' (Employment Equality Acts 1998–2015). The Disability Act 2005 defines 'disability', albeit in a different context, as '[...] a substantial restriction in the capacity of the person to carry on a profession, business or occupation [...] by reason of an enduring physical [or] sensory [...] impairment'.

While Irish legislation makes no reference to chronic illness or temporary sickness, the equality authorities make it clear that the provision relating to disability in the Employment Equality Acts must be given a broad definition and scope of application. For example, frequent periods of sick leave can illustrate that the sufferer has a 'disability' for the purposes of the Acts, as determined in the case of *Fernandez v Cable and Wireless*. Both asthma and irritable bowel syndrome, for example, have been held to be disabilities on the basis that they are 'malfunctions [...] of a part of a person's body', as set out in *Civil Servant v. Office of Civil Service*.

In other relevant jurisdictions, such as in English law, disability exists where 'a person [...] has a physical or mental impairment, and the impairment has a substantial and long-term adverse effect on [the person's] ability to carry out normal day-to-day activities' (Equality Act 2010). The effect of the impairment is 'long-term' if it lasts, or is expected to last, at least twelve months. The impairment is deemed to affect the ability of the person concerned to carry out normal day-to-day activities if it affects any of the following: mobility; physical co-ordination; ability to lift or carry; speech, hearing or eyesight; or ability to concentrate.

The standards set out in Irish Law (and in English law) for determining disability involve assessments of fact. It is not necessarily the impairment, therefore, that is the determining factor in ascertaining disability. It is the actual effect on the individual. Migraine can therefore count as a disability if the adverse effect on the individual concerned is substantial and long-term, affecting them in carrying out normal day-to-day activities. While this is not necessarily the case in every EU Member State, where the employment rights available are more uncertain, the broad definition of 'disability' set out in Irish law certainly makes it possible that the provisions of the EU Directive, as transposed by the Employment Equality Acts 1998–2015, can be applied to those who are affected in their workplace by the symptoms of migraine.

LEGAL PROTECTION AVAILABLE FOR CHRONIC MIGRAINE SUFFERERS

If the chronic migraine sufferer can be classified as 'disabled', even possibly temporarily so, for the purposes of the Equal Treatment Directive and the Employment Equality Acts, then it is clear that 'the provision of measures to accommodate [their] needs at the workplace [is required as it is recognised that this] plays an important role in combating discrimination on grounds of disability'. It is important to note that the legislation goes on to say that the law 'does not require the recruitment, promotion, maintenance in employment or training of an individual who is not competent, capable and available to perform the essential functions of the post concerned or to undergo the relevant training, without prejudice to the obligation to provide reasonable accommodation for people with disabilities'.

However, it is further stated that 'appropriate measures should be provided', i.e. effective and practical measures to adapt the workplace to the disability, for example:

o   Adapting premises and equipment.
o   Patterns of working time.
o   The distribution of tasks.
o   The provision of training or integration resources.

If the person is capable of doing the job, and has been employed to do the job, then reasonable accommodation should be made in the workplace to facilitate their carrying out of the tasks related to the job.

Potentially, therefore, the key provision of the legislation for migraine sufferers is set out in Article 5 of the Directive, and Section 16 of the Irish Act. The Directive states that 'in order to guarantee compliance with the principle of equal treatment in relation to persons with disabilities, reasonable accommodation shall be provided [including] that employers shall take appropriate measures, where needed in a particular case, to enable a person with a disability to have access to, participate in, or advance in employment, or to undergo training, unless such measures would impose a disproportionate burden on the employer'.

The Directive makes it clear that employers, both public and private, must take appropriate measures, within their budgets, to facilitate those who suffer from a disability. Accommodation should, therefore, be made in the workplace to ensure that the chances of the migraineur suffering an attack, or repeated attacks, is minimised. Employers are obliged to make a 'reasonable adjustment' in the circumstances.

Section 16(3) of the Employment Equality Acts provides that '[a]n employer shall do all that is reasonable to accommodate the needs of a person who has a disability by providing special treatment or facilities [that enable the employee to carry out his or her duties]. Refusal to provide this special treatment or facilities is deemed to be unreasonable '[...] unless such provision would give rise to a cost, other than a nominal cost, to the employer'.

The EU Directive further seeks to facilitate consultation between interested parties on how best to protect employers, and the employees for whom these accommodations need to be made. Adequate measures should be taken between social partners to foster equal treatment, including through the monitoring of workplace practices, collective agreements and codes of conduct. Member States should also encourage dialogue with appropriate non-governmental organisations which have a legitimate interest in contributing to the fight against discrimination and the facilitation of appropriate employment environments.

OTHER RELEVANT LEGAL INSTRUMENTS AND TEXTS

Other legal texts lend weight to the obligation imposed to ensure that those classified as suffering from a disability receive set minimum levels of protection. For example, the Charter of Fundamental Rights of the European Union states that 'any discrimination based on any ground such as [...] disability [...] shall be prohibited'. The Charter now has full legal status within EU Law and therefore applies in Ireland also.

In addition to this, the Community Charter of the Fundamental Social Rights of Workers states that 'all disabled persons, whatever the origin and nature of their disablement, must be entitled to additional concrete measures aimed at improving their social and professional integration'. The need, and obligation, to protect those suffering from a debilitating condition that affects the ability to work properly is clearly provided for, not just in the terms of the Equal Treatment Directive and the Employment Equality Acts, but also in other, more general provisions operating in EU law, such as the Charter of Fundamental Rights and the Charter of Social Rights.

INTERNATIONAL MEASURES

International organisations, such as the World Health Organisation (WHO), recognise that headache disorders such as migraine impose pain and disability on people throughout the world. The United Nations has recognised the need to make reasonable accommodation where required in the Convention on the Rights of Persons with Disabilities (Ireland was amongst the first EU Member States to sign the Convention, but it is amongst the last to ratify it). Disorders such as chronic migraine are clearly considered 'disabilities' in the international arena, worthy of being accorded the protection available under existing equality and anti-discrimination provisions.

If chronic migraine is to be widely considered as a 'disability', bringing those who suffer from it within the scope of existing employment protection laws in Ireland, then the need to ensure that these international conventions are also applied to migraineurs exists. Failure to recognise debilitating transitory conditions results in a failure to adhere to the most generally applicable and fundamentally important of international obligations, such as those arising under the terms of the United Nations Universal Declaration of Human Rights and also the Conventions of the International Labour Organisation, such as that on Discrimination (Employment and Occupation) in 1958.

CONCLUDING REMARKS AND FUTURE DEVELOPMENTS

An examination into the current status of chronic migraine sufferers under EU and Irish employment equality laws suggests the following:

o Satisfactory legal provisions do exist for those suffering from 'disabilities'.
o Primarily, the obligation on employers to make 'reasonable adjustments' for those who are impaired in their work presents an

opportunity to both accommodate migraineurs in the workplace and minimise any economic or productivity losses arising out of their condition.

The main impediment to ensuring that these provisions are properly implemented and applied is the absence of any standardised legal definition of 'disability', as applicable to migraineurs.

At present, EU Member States are relatively free to determine who is protected under equality laws on the basis of disability. This leads to an inconsistent application of the Equal Treatment Directive across the EU. As a result, workers in some Member States are given less protection than that which is available elsewhere. However, the level of protection available under Irish application of the relevant EU laws is relatively high. 'Disability' is defined in Irish law in a broad sense, offering scope for certain migraineurs to be protected and accommodated under the Employment Equality Acts.

Irish law clearly recognises that the actual *effect* on the individual, rather than the condition suffered, is central to determining who should be protected under the Employment Equality Acts. It is the nature of the migraine and the effect that it has on the employee, as well as the cost to the employer, that determines whether, and to what extent, accommodation or allowances must be made.

Further support for the position of migraineurs in the workplace exists in the documents and position of key international organisations, such as the World Health Organisation, who have made it clear that migraine is a disability. Those suffering from this condition in a manner that affects their day-to-day activities, even on a transitory basis, should therefore be covered by the existing employment equality laws.

Strong provision is made in existing legislation, both Irish and European Union, to ensure that employers are only obliged to make those accommodations that do not have an unreasonable or significant adverse effect on their resources. What is required, therefore, is a recognition of debilitating conditions through making reasonable adjustments to working practices and environment that do not have a significant adverse impact on the employer.

Employers are also entitled under Section 35 of the Employment Equality Acts to offer lower rates of pay to employees with a disability – but only where the disability affects the employee's productivity or ability to carry out all aspects of the job.

Making these reasonable adjustments can be achieved through consultation with individual employees, their collective representatives and interested non-governmental organisations or independent public bodies, such as the Irish Human Rights and Equality Commission, the Migraine Association of Ireland and the European Headache Alliance. The Treaty on the Functioning of the European Union, the Equal Treatment Directive and the Conventions of the International Labour Organisation all advocate this approach.

Where a migraineur does not believe that reasonable accommodation has been made in the workplace to account for his or her condition, a complaint must be lodged within six months of this refusal, or some other discriminatory act. This complaint should now be made to the Workplace Relations Commission. It is entirely unlawful under the Employment Equality Acts for an employer to take any action against an employee who makes such a complaint.

Finally, and following on from the aims of the Global Campaign to Reduce the Burden of Headache, awareness needs to be raised amongst legislators, employers and society generally about the debilitating nature of chronic migraine. This is vital to ensuring that the key provisions of existing employment laws are properly implemented at EU, national and local levels, and are provided for those affected in their work from the debilitating effects of conditions such as migraine.

11

SOME TIPS FOR LIVING WITH MIGRAINE

Migraine Association of Ireland Helpline Team

MIGRAINE AND LIFE

We now know that migraine is far more than just pain and weird peripheral visions. Sufferers go through a whole gamut of symptoms, many of which affect their lives equally as badly as the pain. To try to help sufferers cope with their disorder, and to inform those who live and work around them, this final chapter is devoted to tips to help get the most out of life.

If you suffer from migraine, the first thing you need to do is educate yourself. By reading this book, you've already begun that journey. Understanding your own condition and educating your family, friends and colleagues alike, is the way forward. With the right information, support, treatment and understanding, the majority of migraineurs can bring their condition under control, reducing the frequency and severity of attacks, thereby living a full life.

DAY-TO-DAY LIFE

Here are some tips that may help you through:

o Take responsibility and learn about your condition.
o Keep a migraine diary to try to identify your triggers or pattern of attacks.

o Learn to recognise your symptoms so that you will know when an attack is about to happen.
o Talk to your GP about management and treatment plans.
o Have your medication handy at all times.
o Stick to regular eating and sleeping patterns – the migraine brain likes routine.
o Make time for relaxation and regular light exercise.
o Drink plenty of water.
o Reduce stress as much as possible.
o Don't be afraid to ask for help if you need it – it's a good idea to have one person who understands the condition to call on should the need arise.
o Educate your boss and colleagues in work; tell your teachers in school and college.

MIGRAINE AND WORK

Migraine in work can be a daunting prospect. Many sufferers are reluctant to tell their colleagues or boss, but telling them could be the difference between having a fulfilling career or not. Here are a few tips for employees who suffer from migraine and find it affecting their work:

o Take regular breaks, especially from computer screens and stressful situations.
o Try to make your working environment as comfortable as possible.
o Do regular exercises to avoid stiffness and tension.
o Keep a fan nearby or ask to change your desk to one near a window.
o If you work outdoors a lot or drive, make sure you have a proper pair of *polarised* sunglasses and/or a pair of wrap-around shades.
o If you drive around the country, plan well and try to make sure you have plenty of time and are not under pressure to make a meeting.
o While driving, recognise early symptoms so that you can pull in and take your medication, then if necessary and possible, find a safe place and have a rest or a sleep in the car.

WHAT CAN I DO AS AN EMPLOYER?

- o Educate yourself and your staff.
- o Let your staff know that you are open to them coming to you about health problems and be supportive to those who do.
- o Learn the signs and symptoms of migraine.
- o Contact the MAI for help and information.
- o Come to any of our free Migraine Events.
- o Be tolerant of someone who seems to have slowed down; don't assume that because someone looks well, they feel fine.
- o Install and maintain a good lighting system which is as near to natural daylight as possible.
- o Try to keep noise levels to a minimum.
- o Provide computer screens with a low flicker rate, or non-flickering screens.
- o Design or install ergonomic workstations.
- o Be aware of patterns in carpeting or decor you might be having done, such as zigzag lines, houndstooth pattern.
- o Have readily available drinking water.
- o Organise wellness days for your staff.
- o Consider allowing flexible working hours.
- o Provide a darkened area or rest room for staff.
- o Provide stress management training.
- o Allow breaks as often as necessary for food and medication.
- o Let people know that if they are unwell, they are not expected to show up for work until they feel that they can.

With the help of informed and sympathetic colleagues you can participate fully in a rewarding working life.

MIGRAINE AND EXAMS

Over 100,000 children in Ireland suffer from migraine and it can manifest differently in a child than in an adult. The stress during exam time can have a detrimental effect on students who suffer from migraine.

To allow for students with disabilities, the State Examinations Commission (SEC) has devised Reasonable Accommodations (covered in Chapter 1). By taking the disability into account, these Reasonable Accommodations take some of the pressure off, giving the student the same opportunity as anyone who doesn't suffer from migraine.

SCHOOL

There are several things that the school can do to take some exam pressure off students with migraine before approaching the SEC. You can discuss these prior to the exams and most schools are accommodating. The student should provide a letter from their GP/neurologist stating that they suffer from migraine. The school may then allow:

o Breaks or time to rest during an exam – time taken for breaks may be added to the end of each exam period up to a maximum of twenty minutes.
o Medicine, food or drinks to be taken into the exam centre.
o The student to get up and move around in the exam centre.
o The use of a special desk or chair if necessary.

There may be other things schools are prepared to do, but they must be discussed well in advance of the exams.

PARENTS

Parents can play a huge part in helping their child through exams with the least amount of pressure and worry. The most important thing you can do for your child is to let them know that you support them regardless of the results of their exams. Other things to bear in mind are:

o Stay calm and relaxed, and be supportive and encouraging. Think back to what you went through when you sat your own exams.

o If they're having difficulty studying, try to break their work into more manageable parts and don't worry if a migraine causes them to miss an evening here or there.

o Watch for changes in behaviour or signs that the pressure may be getting too much for them. Encourage them to talk to you.

o Make sure that they stick to their normal routine as much as possible; this is particularly important for the migraine brain.

o Be realistic with your child. The exams are important, yes, but they are not the be-all and end-all of life.

TEACHERS

Teachers are very important for students who suffer from migraine. They can fill a gap when parents can't be there:

o Make yourself fully aware of students' problems and disabilities and be encouraging.

o Watch for signs of stress, depression and anxiety.

o Keep your own stress levels to a minimum.

o Introduce Mindfulness or another relaxation technique into the classroom.

o Make sure you know what to do in the case of a migraine attack.

o If possible, remove the student to a dark, quiet room to reduce the severity of the attack. Sometimes a short sleep or cold pack can help get them back into the classroom quickly.

o Make sure someone stays with or near them until the attack subsides or if necessary call the parents and send the child home.

o Let the students know you are there to support them and that they can come to you should they need to.

o Allow for extra breaks in class or during a study period, especially if they're in front of a computer screen for long intervals.

ON THE DAY OF THE EXAM

If you're a teacher who happens to be supervising the sitting of the exam:

o   Make sure you're aware of any accommodations the school has granted to a student and let the student know that it's okay if they need to use these accommodations.
o   Be prepared to let them take breaks and give them the added time if necessary. Have extra water nearby in case the student needs it.
o   If they need to have a short snack or to take medications allow them the time to do this.

STUDENTS

We hope that these tips will help you to sail through your exams to get on with your exciting new life after school.

o   Stay calm as much as possible.
o   Organise your study time well in advance to help you to reduce your own stress. Make a revision timetable to suit you.
o   Talk about the Reasonable Accommodations. Discuss with your parents, teacher and school what they might be able to do to help.
o   If you are not happy with how anyone has responded to your condition, feel free to contact us. We can send information for teachers and parents that might help them to help you.
o   Study in a place and environment that suits you.
o   Ask for help when you need to. No matter what kind you need, don't be afraid to ask.
o   Studying in itself can be stressful and takes quite a lot of energy. Make sure you stick to your usual routine as much as possible.
o   Take regular breaks and eat regular meals. Try to avoid triggers and don't be afraid to take a longer break than normal if you're not feeling well.

o Be careful not to skip meals in order to keep studying and make sure you have plenty of water.

o Make sure you go to bed at the same time each night. Staying up late to study is a sure-fire way of triggering a migraine. Sleep is important for your memory and concentration.

o Try to distract yourself from studying every now and then. If you play sports, go training. If you like walking or running, go out and get some fresh air.

o If you are feeling stressed, tell someone, even if it's only a friend. If you don't feel comfortable about talking to people you know, then call the ISPCC Support Line on (01) 676 7960 from Monday to Friday between 9 a.m. and 5 p.m.

o Exams are important and it's great to get good results, but not getting the result you want is not the end of the world. There are always options. There are other places to go for help, and if you don't get enough points for your first choice college course, then there are organisations like Access College or Ahead who might be able to help you.

MIGRAINE AND HOLIDAYS

After all the exams are over, it's time for holidays, but as a migraine sufferer you're forever waiting for that next attack. Here are some tips which may help combat that holiday migraine.

ROUTINE

o Stick to your routine on holiday as much as possible. Try to get up, eat and sleep at the same time as usual.

o Gradually change your routine to take account of local time.

o Bring an extra watch and leave it on Irish time to help you figure out when to do things.

STRESS LESS

- If possible, take the two days before your holiday off.
- Do as much preparation as possible in the weeks coming up to the holiday and avoid leaving everything until the last minute.

MEDICATION

- Make sure you have all your medication with you. Some countries require you to bring your prescriptions as well, so make sure you have them packed too.
- Ask the doctor for a short note explaining your need for your medication. It will help if you need added medication, to see a GP abroad or for customs.
- Ask your doctor for an extra prescription or medication if you'll be away for a while.
- If you're bringing extra medication, don't keep it all in one bag in case one gets accidentally sent to the wrong location.
- If you are going to a foreign country, it's a good idea to check out where the local health/medical centre/GP is and if anyone there speaks your language.
- Check to see if that country has a national migraine organisation which might give you information on where to go for help.
- Keep a Migraine Identity Card on you so you can hand to a person should a severe attack occur and you can't communicate.

AIRPORT

- Many airports have a quiet area, prayer room or chapel, which are normally darker than the rest of the airport and much quieter. All airports ban the use of mobile phones in these areas.
- Don't be afraid to ask for help from the airport police or staff if you need it.
- If you're worried about being searched and the hassle of taking

off your shoes and opening out your bags, be ready. Wear shoes or sandals that can be easily slipped off and on, only put essentials in your hand luggage and keep your pockets free if possible.

o For information on facilities at your destination or returning airport, see their individual airport websites.

TRAVEL

o Talk to your doctor beforehand about medication or alternative treatments for motion sickness.
o Keep hydrated: bring water with you everywhere.
o If you're driving down the country with children in the car, bring games, books or DVDs to occupy them when you are stuck in traffic.
o Let plenty of air into the car, even if it's not that warm.
o Give yourself sufficient time to get there so you're not rushing, that way even being stuck in traffic won't be too stressful.
o Break your journey, even if it's not too long a drive, stop at a town or rest stop, get out, stretch your legs, have a bite to eat and relax for a while.
o If travelling on a long-haul flight or train journey, don't be afraid to get up, stretch a bit and walk about the place if possible.
o Ask for an aisle seat so that you don't have to climb across sleeping passengers to get out of your seat or to get access to the toilet.
o Consider trying some travel aids: some can help with nausea and others reduce the noise and help with air pressure.

FOOD

o Be aware of food triggers and try to check the ingredients on menus, especially if it's not the kind of food you would normally eat.
o Tell your hotel, tour operator or the airline in advance.
o Drink plenty of water and make sure you have access to water, especially in a hot climate.

RELAX

- o Try to relax as much as possible. Whether you're in Spain, Italy or here in Ireland, take a 'siesta' in the afternoon if you feel the need.
- o You're on holiday, it's your time, and so make sure you factor in some 'me time'.
- o Discuss this with family and friends before you go so that it can be planned for and no one will be disappointed if you're not on a trip or activity.

ACTIVITIES

- o If you're an active person and plan on skiing, walking, hiking, or surfing, don't overexert yourself. Know your limits.
- o Wind down slowly. Try to avoid the sudden stop, as the 'let-down headache' can be painful.
- o Keep your medication on you for handiness.
- o Wear protective sunglasses. Polarised lenses reduce the glare and wrap-around shades block the sun from sneaking in the corners of your eyes.
- o Make a packing checklist for days out, for example hat, sunglasses, sun cream, water, medication, money and emergency contact phone numbers. Keep everything you need ready in a bag.

SIGHTSEEING

- o If you're rushing to see too many things in too little time it can add unwanted stress, so try to prioritise the most important sights and take your time. It is better to miss one or two sights and enjoy the rest without a migraine than to rush around, trigger a migraine and miss them all, as well as the rest of the holiday.

For further information see www.migraine.ie, or call our helpline – 1850 200 378.

SOURCES

General tips
o https://migraine.com
o http://www.migraine.org.uk

Exam tips:
o https://www.examinations.ie/?l=en&mc=ca&sc=ra
o http://ie.reachout.com/inform-yourself/money-work-and-study/
  exams/managing-exam-stress
o http://www.ispcc.ie

Holiday tips
o http://www.vestibular.org
o http://www.menieres.org.uk
o http://www.hse.ie/eng/services/list/1/schemes/EHIC

Work tips
o http://www.hsa.ie/eng/Publications_and_Forms/Publications/
  Latest_Publications/Ergonomics_-_Good_Practice_in_the_
  Irish_Workplace.64413.shortcut.html

GLOSSARY

A

Abdominal Migraine
Symptoms such as stomach ache, loss of appetite, nausea and vomiting without headache, which is the way migraine in children can manifest itself.

Acute Treatment
Medicine to provide relief.

Allodynia
Pain caused by something that wouldn't usually cause pain.

Analgesics
Painkillers such as paracetamol.

Anti-emetics
Drugs taken to prevent nausea or vomiting.

Antioxidant Activity
Actions of substances which inhibit certain compounds.

Aneurysm
Excessive dilatation of the wall of an artery.

Aphasia
Inability or impaired ability to understand or produce speech.

Arnold–Chiari Malformation
A particular malformation present at birth involving some of the brain descending out of the skull. It is associated with spina bifida.

B

Barometric Pressure
Atmospheric pressure.

Basilar Migraine
Rare form of migraine.

Benign
   Not malignant.

Beta Blockers
   Class of drugs to prevent migraine.

Bilateral Location
   The pain is in both sides of the head.

Biochemical Individuality
   The different ways that people respond to chemicals.

Biofeedback
   A treatment technique in which people are trained using technology
   to control their bodies by using signals from their bodies. The person
   is connected to electrical sensors that receive information (feedback)
   about their bodies (bio).

Botulinum Toxin
   Botox.

C

Cerebral
   Brain.

Cerebral Aneurysm
   A dilatation in the wall of an artery supplying the brain.

Cervicogenic Headaches
   Headaches caused by neck disorder or lesion.

Chronic
   Persistent over time.

Chronic Migraine
   More than fifteen days per month.

Clinical Examination
   Physical or medical examination.

Co-morbid
   The greater then coincidental existence of two conditions occurring in
   the same individual.

CT Scan
   A special radiological investigation to image the brain.

Cutaneous Allodynia
   The perception of pain from a normal stimulus such as light touch, e.g.
   combing the hair.

D

Demographic Features
  Statistical segments of the population.

Diagnosis
  Identifying a disease, illness or problem.

Disability
  A substantial restriction in the capacity of the person to carry on a profession, business or occupation.

Dispensing
  Preparation and provision of prescribed drugs.

Dura
  Tough outermost membrane surrounding the brain and spinal cord.

E

European Headache Alliance
  Umbrella organisation of headache patient groups across Europe.

Equal Treatment Directive
  European Union directive protecting workers' rights.

G

Greater Occipital Nerve
  A cranial nerve that transmits painful sensory information from the scalp at the top of the head.

H

Hemiplegia
  One-sided paralysis.

Hemiplegic Migraine
  A rare but severe form of migraine where temporary paralysis occurs, usually on one side of the body (hemi = half).

Homonymous Visual Disturbance
  Loss of vision towards one side in each eye but it is the result of disturbance in the brain and not in the eyes.

I

Idiopathic
Cause uncertain or unknown.

Imaging Technology
Technology which shows us the brain in action.

Intracranial
Inside the skull.

Intracranial Hypertension
Abnormally high pressure inside the skull.

M

Ménière's Disease
A disorder of the inner ear.

Meninges
The three membranes or 'skins' that cover the brain and spinal cord.

Metabolic Processes
Activity in the cells and tissues during which energy is released.

MRI
Magnetic Resonance Imaging is a noninvasive technological diagnostic tool which provides images of the brain.

Multimodal Therapy
The combination of at least two or more treatment options in managing an illness.

N

Negative Double Blind Study
A study in which nobody at all knows who is taking the 'real' drug or the 'fake', or placebo, drug.

Neural Networking
A proposed system of interconnecting brain cells which attempts to explain brain function, e.g. memory.

Neurobiofeedback
A form of biofeedback or training for the brain using technology which shows the brain working.

Neurological Disorder
> Brain and nervous system disorder.

Neuromodulatory Agents
> Agents that change nerve activity through electrical stimulation.

Neuropeptides
> Small molecules which are released from nerve terminals during a migraine attack.

Neuromodulatory Therapies
> A substance released from a nerve that alters the activity of other nerves.

Non-pharmacological Management Techniques
> Non-drug ways or ways of helping other than with medication.

O

Occipital Nerve
> The nerve which transmits sensory information from the back of the head to the brain.

Ophthalmoplegic Migraines (also known as Ocular Migraine)
> A rare form of migraine headache.

P

Palpation
> A form of examination using the palm of the hand as part of the physical examination to aid diagnosis.

Paroxysmal Hemicranias
> Multiple severe, short headache attacks affecting only one side of the cranium.

Pathogenesis
> The origin and development of a disease.

Pathophysiology
> The study of changes that occur in the body as a result of disease.

Patterned Visual Stimuli
> Pictures that provoke a response in a person.

Phonophobia
> Sensitive to or unable to tolerate noise.

Photophobia
> Sensitive to or unable to tolerate light.

Positron Emission Tomography (PET)
> Imaging test that helps reveal how tissues and organs are functioning by using a 'tracer' or drug to show this activity.

Post-Traumatic Headaches
> Headaches that begin within one week following a head injury.

Premonitory symptoms
> Warning signs.

Presenting Symptom
> Main complaint or reason for seeking treatment.

Prophylactic or Prophylaxis
> Preventative.

Prophylactic Therapy
> Preventative treatment.

Prevalance
> The percentage of a population that is affected with a given disease at a given time.

Prodromal
> Initial onset time of an attack.

Prophylaxis
> Prophylactic therapy.

Psychological Society of Ireland (PSI)
> The learned and professional body for Psychology in the Republic of Ireland. See www.psihq.ie.

Psychosocial stressors
> Stress when we perceive that the demands on us outweigh our capacity to deal with them.

R

Reasonable Accommodation
> Under the Equal Status Act, educational institutions are required to do all that is reasonably in their power to support students with disability.

Reasonable Accommodation in Exams
> Modifications in how a test is administered while not compromising the integrity of the examination system. See www.examinations.ie for details.

Rebound Headache

Headache caused by ongoing medication overuse for pain relief of headache.

Refractory Headaches

Headaches that are resistant to treatment.

Reye's Syndrome

A rare but serious condition that most often affects children and teen-agers recovering from a viral infection, most commonly the flu or chickenpox.

S

Sensory Disturbance

Disruption of sensory information being transmitted to the brain.

Serotonin Receptors

Specific sites of action in nerve cells in the brain where serotonin, a chemical, is active.

Sjaastad Syndrome

A rare form of one-sided headache.

T

Thunderclap Headache

A severe, sudden-onset headache which reaches maximum intensity within one minute.

Transcranial Electrical Stimulation

Electrical stimulation through the skull.

Transcutaneous Nerve Stimulation

Stimulation of nerves through the skin.

Tricyclic Anti-depressants

A group of drugs used in the prevention of headaches.

Trigeminal Ganglion

The location of nerve cells which transmit sensory/painful information from the front and side of the head.

Triptan Drugs

A specific group of anti-migraine therapies to provide relief from an attack.

U

Unilateral Paraesthesias
   One-sided tingling, pins and needles and/or numbness.

Unilateral Vestibular Loss
   When one side of the vestibular system or inner ear system concerned
   with balance is impaired.

V

Vagal
   A nerve in the body which controls numerous functions such as secre-
   tion of mucous and production of tears.

Vascular System
   Relating to blood vessels.

Vestibulopathies
   Medical conditions caused by abnormal functioning of the vestibular
   (hearing) mechanisms.

Visceral
   The gut.

Vestibular Symptoms
   Symptoms caused by disruption in the hearing apparatus, e.g. poor balance, buzzing in the ears and impaired hearing.

Visual Disturbance
   Alteration in an individual's vision.

W

WHO
   World Health Organisation.

Workplace Relations Commission (WRC)
   An independent, statutory body whose core services include the inspec-
   tion of employment rights compliance, the provision of information,
   the processing of employment agency and protection of young persons'
   (employment) licences and the provision of mediation, conciliation,
   facilitation and advisory services.